Overcoming Fear

Deborah Ward is a writer and editor whose passion for personal growth and psychology has led to the publication of numerous feature articles for a variety of print and online magazines. With a desire to nurture the personal development, self-esteem and potential of others, she also writes a regular blog for *Psychology Today* magazine called Sense and Sensitivity, on the subject of coping with high sensitivity. Deborah's creative interests also include writing fiction. She has published numerous short stories and is currently also working on a novel. Through her writing, Deborah strives to provide the clarity and compassion to inspire others to be their true selves and to shed light on issues which are so often hidden in darkness.

D0351675

467 471 05 7

Overcoming Common Problems Series

Selected titles

A full list of titles is available from Sheldon Press,
36 Causton Street, London SW1P 4ST and on our website at
www.sheldonpress.co.uk

Breast Cancer: Your treatment choices
Dr Terry Priestman

Cider Vinegar
Margaret Hills

Coeliac Disease: What you need to know
Alex Gazzola

**Coping Successfully with Chronic Illness:
Your healing plan**
Neville Shone

Coping Successfully with Shyness
Margaret Oakes, Professor Robert Bor
and Dr Carina Eriksen

Coping with Anaemia
Dr Tom Smith

Coping with Difficult Families
Dr Jane McGregor and Tim McGregor

Coping with Drug Problems in the Family
Lucy Jolin

Coping with Eating Disorders and Body Image
Christine Craggs-Hinton

Coping with Epilepsy
Dr Pamela Crawford and Fiona Marshall

Coping with Gout
Christine Craggs-Hinton

Coping with Liver Disease
Mark Greener

Coping with Obsessive Compulsive Disorder
Professor Kevin Gournay, Rachel Piper
and Professor Paul Rogers

Coping with Schizophrenia
Professor Kevin Gournay and Debbie Robson

Depressive Illness: The Curse of the Strong
Dr Tim Cantopher

The Diabetes Healing Diet
Mark Greener and Christine Craggs-Hinton

Dying for a Drink
Dr Tim Cantopher

**The Empathy Trap: Understanding Antisocial
Personalities**
Dr Jane McGregor and Tim McGregor

**Epilepsy: Complementary and alternative
treatments**
Dr Sallie Baxendale

Fibromyalgia: Your Treatment Guide
Christine Craggs-Hinton

Hay Fever: How to beat it
Dr Paul Carson

The Heart Attack Survival Guide
Mark Greener

Helping Elderly Relatives
Jill Eckersley

The Holistic Health Handbook
Mark Greener

How to Come Out of Your Comfort Zone
Dr Windy Dryden

How to Eat Well When You Have Cancer
Jane Freeman

How to Stop Worrying
Dr Frank Tallis

The Irritable Bowel Diet Book
Rosemary Nicol

Living with Complicated Grief
Professor Craig A. White

Living with IBS
Nuno Ferreira and David T. Gillanders

**Making Sense of Trauma: How to tell
your story**
Dr Nigel C. Hunt and Dr Sue McHale

Overcoming Fear: With mindfulness
Deborah Ward

Overcoming Loneliness
Alice Muir

The Panic Workbook
Dr Carina Eriksen, Professor Robert Bor
and Margaret Oakes

**Physical Intelligence: How to take charge
of your weight**
Dr Tom Smith

The Self-Esteem Journal
Alison Waines

**Transforming Eight Deadly Emotions
into Healthy Ones**
Dr Windy Dryden

Treating Arthritis: The drug-free way
Margaret Hills and Christine Horner

Treating Arthritis: The supplements guide
Julia Davies

**When Someone You Love Has Depression:
A handbook for family and friends**
Barbara Baker

Overcoming Common Problems

Overcoming Fear

With mindfulness

DEBORAH WARD

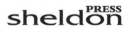

First published in Great Britain in 2013

Sheldon Press
36 Causton Street
London SW1P 4ST
www.sheldonpress.co.uk

The author and publisher have made every effort to ensure that the external
website and email addresses included in this book are correct and up to date at the
time of going to press. The author and publisher are not responsible for the content,
quality or continuing accessibility of the sites.

British Library Cataloguing-in-Publication Data
A catalogue record for this book is available from the British Library

ISBN 978-1-84709-286-1
eBook ISBN 978-1-84709-287-8

Typeset by Caroline Waldron, Wirral, Cheshire
First printed in Great Britain by Ashford Colour Press
Subsequently digitally printed in Great Britain

Produced on paper from sustainable forests

Contents

Love is what we are born with. Fear is what we learn.

Marianne Williamson

Action conquers fear.

Peter Nivio Zarlenga

He who is not everyday conquering some fear
has not learned the secret of life.

Ralph Waldo Emerson

Introduction

Sylvia had always known what it was like to live with fear. When she was growing up, her parents often argued. Her father would get angry and drink too much while her mother hid in the bedroom, but Sylvia could hear her crying as the doors kept slamming. It wasn't until she had become an adult herself and moved out that they finally got a divorce. By then, Sylvia was in a relationship of her own with a kind and intelligent young man, but she often found herself feeling anxious around him. Whenever he offered to drive her to work or when he bought her a gift, she felt her heart pounding and her hands begin to sweat. She had no idea why she felt this way. But when he asked her to move in together, she felt so afraid that she began to shake all over. All she wanted to do was run away. And so she told him that their relationship had to end.

What was Sylvia afraid of? Was she afraid of commitment? Or was it something she was not even aware of, something that had nothing to do with her boyfriend? Sylvia's experiences with relationships as a child had not been very positive and so she learned early on to be afraid of them. To her, they only made people unhappy. And while she was aware of the way she felt, she was completely unaware of the real cause of that fear or what she could do about it. She felt fearful around her boyfriend, so it made sense to blame him for her feelings. She coped with her fear by avoiding it, but it never went away.

The feeling of fear is familiar to everyone, whether it's a fear of commitment, a fear of failure, a fear of change or a fear of rejection. While fear is a common and natural response, it can also become debilitating, affecting our ability to sleep and work, to do the things we want to do and to enjoy healthy relationships; ultimately it affects our health, preventing us from living lives of joy and peace and from becoming the people we were meant to be.

Part 1 of this book will aim to make you more aware of your own subconscious fears and the ways they direct your choices and attitudes to life. We'll look at the causes of fear, as well as common situations that make us feel fearful and conditions that can trigger our fears. We will also address the kind of person who is, due to temperament, upbringing or biology, more predisposed to fear.

In Part 2, we will discover the ways that mindfulness can help you to overcome fear. By encouraging you to focus on the present moment and develop your awareness, mindfulness can help you to move your thoughts from your unconscious to your conscious mind and to let them go so that you can release the fear those thoughts generate. This section will also explore mindfulness techniques such as mindful eating and mindful walking, meditation, yoga and journalling. We'll look at the ways in which mindfulness can help you overcome fear in your relationships and finally we will address work and creativity, and the ways in which mindfulness can help lead you to your dreams.

The difficulty in overcoming our fears is often simply to know that they exist, how they are affecting us and what to do about them. Since many of our fears are rooted deep in our earliest experiences they are often below our conscious awareness, and so we go through our lives, day after day, feeling the effects of fear in ourselves and our bodies, in our career choices and in our relationships. Many of us attempt to cope with these unpleasant feelings by avoiding them, either with alcohol, drugs, smoking or food, or by avoiding situations, people or the feelings that are causing the distress. We live our lives on 'autopilot', never really making conscious choices that will lead us to the life we really want to live.

What is fear?

Fear is a physiological response to our perception of danger. Whether we are about to make a speech or we are staring into the eyes of a Bengal tiger, our biological reaction is the same. Under stress, our body releases hormones and prepares us for 'fight or flight'. Symptoms like muscle tension, increased heart rate and shortness of breath are all stress responses to danger. Some other common symptoms of fear include:

- Sweating
- Upset stomach
- Lack of concentration
- Feeling paralysed
- Loss of appetite
- Dry mouth.

Fear can also make you feel edgy and irritable, unable to concentrate and panicked or upset, causing you to desperately seek reassurance and comfort from others. This in turn can create low self-esteem, lower your confidence and trigger feelings of hopelessness, inability to cope, difficulty making decisions, loneliness, withdrawal, frustration, confusion and depression. You may find yourself biting your nails, grinding your teeth or avoiding certain situations.

Fear will also affect your decisions, often without your conscious awareness of it. Fear will make you stay in a situation or a job where you are unhappy because you are too afraid to leave. It will cause you to try to hold on to people or relationships that are no longer working, fearing that you will be alone or rejected or unable to cope on your own. You may feel that it is not worth trying to go for your dreams because you are not worth the effort or that you do not have the talent. All of these thoughts are the consequences of fear, and the effects on your life can be devastating.

Anxiety can often be confused with fear, and they can be hard to distinguish. According to experts, both fear and anxiety are triggered by a threat, either real or imagined, and produce a physiological arousal. But where anxiety puts you on alert to danger, fear drives you to protect yourself in some way. However, fear and anxiety are related because fear can cause us to feel anxious and anxiety can make us feel fearful. Eventually, you can start to fear the symptoms of anxiety so much that you begin to experience those symptoms because you are having fearful thoughts.

Fear and anxiety can easily take over our lives if we don't deal with them effectively. If you feel extremely worried, panicked or fearful most of the time, you may have an anxiety disorder. This type of condition includes panic attacks, post-traumatic stress disorder, obsessive–compulsive disorder and phobias. If you think you have an anxiety disorder, consult your doctor so that you can get professional help.

Although the symptoms and feeling of fear can often be very unpleasant, awareness of your own fear response can provide you with essential information about yourself and your world. Fear is not to be repressed, but noticed. The symptoms of fear are warning signals, in essence, alerting you not only to real dangers but also to subconscious needs that are struggling to be met. By facing them and accepting them in this way, they can evolve from being sources of pain, torment and embarrassment to harmless pieces of information, like a red light at a junction, helping to guide you on your way.

What is mindfulness?

Mindfulness is a mind–body practice based on ancient Zen Buddhist meditation techniques, and has been defined as paying attention in a particular way, in the present moment and without judgement, according to Jon Kabat-Zinn, a researcher at the University of Massachusetts Medical School, who brought mindfulness to the mainstream.

Paying attention means more than just noticing or even being aware. It means being purposefully and deliberately aware of what we are doing in the present moment, how it makes us feel, in terms of our senses and our emotions, how our mind is focused on what we are doing and how it becomes unfocused and wandering. Mindfulness means that you recognize when your mind wanders and you purposefully bring your attention back to the present moment.

The problem with letting your mind wander is that your thoughts tend to focus on your worries, cravings and problems – thoughts which in turn generate feelings of anger, sadness, self-pity and depression and consequently stress, pain and illness. Ruminating over these kinds of thoughts does not solve them but instead reinforces the negative feelings associated with them, causing us to feel increasingly worse.

Mindfulness encourages us to focus on the present moment because much of what we worry about is set either in the past or the future. We feel bad about something that has happened or we worry about something that might happen. Mindfulness reminds us that the only moment that is real is the present moment. Thinking about the past or the future isn't wrong, but we need to do so purposefully, so that we are not losing the joy of our present lives. By doing so, especially in mindfulness practices such as meditation and yoga, we can decrease the effect of negative thoughts and create a space for peace and calmness to develop. With practice, mindfulness gives you the chance to slow down, stop the mental chatter and your habitual, automatic reactions and just breathe.

Becoming aware in a non-judgemental way is another key facet of mindfulness. When you notice thoughts or feelings or your own reactions you simply become aware of them and let them go, without judging them as either good or bad. In this way, you face your thoughts and feelings, yourself and others with an attitude of openness, acceptance and compassion.

Fear is a natural part of life, an instinctive survival technique designed to help us escape from danger. But when the danger is only imagined, the effects of fear on our thoughts, feelings and our health can become detrimental. Mindfulness can help you overcome your fear, so that you do not avoid or ignore it but instead become aware of it, so that you can stop living an unconscious, automatic life based on fear, and start to live a life of peace, joy, creativity and love.

Part 1

ABOUT FEAR

1

Causes of fear and anxiety

What causes fear? And why do some people feel it more than others? The frantic pace of modern life can make anyone feel tense. With constant mobile phone calls and emails, as well as traffic jams, job stress and school fees, it is easy for us all to become classic nail-biters. But some people appear more anxious than others and find it harder to cope. Are they just born worriers? Or is there something else that increases the angst for certain types of people?

A tendency to be fearful is usually determined by genes, personality, the environment in which you grew up or a combination of these. For example, British neuroscientist Philip M. Newton says that people carrying the gene that increases the likelihood of them developing post-traumatic stress disorder (PTSD) will still have to experience significant stress before the disorder develops. Researchers at Emory University assert that many factors contribute to the development of PTSD. Patients who have both the gene that predisposes them to PTSD as well as a history of child abuse go on to develop PTSD, suggesting an interaction between genes and environment that can predict the development of the disorder. So you can be predisposed to certain conditions because of your genes, but the addition of environmental conditions, such as stress, will often trigger it.

Even if you do not have a genetic predisposition for fear you can, under enough stress, become anxious or fearful. But that doesn't mean you are destined for a life of struggle. Knowing whether or not you are likely to become fearful under certain conditions will give you the information and awareness you need to take control of the situation and your life.

Genes

We all have a built-in system for coping with danger, which creates symptoms of fear in response. Researchers have discovered a protein called stathmin, present in the amygdala in the brain, which controls the ability to react with appropriate fear to impending danger. Mice without the gene for this protein show abnormally low levels of anxiety in situations that should inspire fear. So it appears that our brains are hard-wired to react with fear to certain situations. But there are individual differences in how this protein and other brain chemicals operate within us, and the degree to which it affects different people.

Harvard psychologist Jerome Kagan believed that people are born with one of two temperaments: inhibited or uninhibited. According to Kagan, an inhibited individual is shy, timid and fearful and an uninhibited person is bold, sociable and outgoing. These temperaments are not only present in people at birth but also, Kagan theorized, predictive of later behaviour in adulthood. Whether or not inhibited types become anxious adults, however, depends on their experiences in their environment. Inhibited children are born with a lower threshold for arousal of various brain regions, wrote Kagan, particularly the amygdala, the area where fear is formed and the region responsible for the production of cortisol, a hormone that is released under stress. When these regions of the brain were stimulated, the inhibited children exhibited signs of anxiety.

Likewise, a study in the journal *Behavioural Neuroscience* has found a link between genes and anxious behaviour. Some people carry a certain gene that regulates the neurotransmitter dopamine and consequently have what researchers call an 'exaggerated startle reflex'. This biochemical condition, say the researchers, explains why some people find it harder to regulate their emotional reaction to arousal. In other words, some people are genetically more sensitive to their environment. This innate sensitivity, when combined with environmental or social factors such as stress or a difficult childhood, can make them more prone to fear and anxiety.

Dr Elaine Aron, author of *The Highly Sensitive Person*, wrote about people who are genetically sensitive to their environment. She found that about 15–20 per cent of the population are what she terms 'highly sensitive people' (HSP), meaning they are very aware of and react intensely to the sensory stimulation around them. The HSP has a sensitive nervous system, a trait that is often inherited. Because of their innate sensitivity, HSPs startle easily and become rattled when they have too much to do. HSPs are very aware of subtleties in their environment and consequently become easily overwhelmed by overstimulation, causing them to respond with symptoms of fear and anxiety. Subtleties in the environment can include any sensory information, such as bright lights, loud noises, strong smells, unusual tastes and coarse fabrics, as well as the feelings and moods of other people. Being around someone who is angry, for example, can move an HSP to tears, as can the honking of a car horn or the flashing of bright lights. Crowds can often become sources of stress for HSPs, not only because of the noise but also the volume of energy generated by large groups of people.

HSPs do not respond to this kind of overstimulation because they are afraid but because they are sensitive to their environment. However, too much stimulation, stress and emotion tends to make HSPs susceptible to feelings of fear and anxiety. They do not fear people or loud noises or crowds, but they can come to fear the feeling of being overwhelmed caused by such stimulation. Additionally, HSPs are often struggling to cope with their own self-doubt, confusion and the need to feel understood and accepted by others, all of which can create an anxious and fearful type of person.

Temperament

After years of collecting data from people with anxiety, anxiety coach Charles Linden revealed that 'our data shows us that anxiety sufferers all share a superior level of creative intellect'.

Sensitive people *need* to be creative as a way of releasing the energy they have absorbed, which would otherwise turn into depression, anxiety or crippling fear. As Pulitzer Prize and Nobel Prize winner Pearl S. Buck wrote:

> The truly creative mind in any field is no more than this: A human creature born abnormally, inhumanly sensitive. To him, a touch is a blow, a sound is a noise, a misfortune is a tragedy, a joy is an ecstasy, a friend is a lover, a lover is a god, and failure is death. Add to this cruelly delicate organism the overpowering necessity to create, create, create, – so that without the creating of music or poetry or books or buildings or something of meaning, his very breath is cut off from him. He must create, must pour out creation. By some strange, unknown, inward urgency he is not really alive unless he is creating.

Many sensitive or gifted individuals have high standards, as well as a low tolerance for mediocrity and frustration. They have an acute awareness of complexities and consequences and a strong need for self-determination, among other characteristics. And while these qualities can give people the drive, organization and focus to help them achieve their goals, they can also create feelings of worry, anxiety and depression, as well as fear, such as the fear of failure or the fear of not living up to others' expectations.

This fear of other people's opinions is one of the common reasons that people feel fear, whether you are sensitive and creative or not. People are often afraid to let anyone else know how they are really feeling. But the efforts involved in keeping your own negative feelings a secret, as well as the isolation it can cause, only exacerbates the situation.

In a recent study in the *Journal of Personality and Social Psychology*, people were shown to judge themselves as more anxious, inhibited and shy than other people. We think that it is only ourselves who have the problem, which in turn makes us feel bad about ourselves and more anxious to hide our fears. We often come to this conclusion because most people are hiding their true feelings, so it only *appears* as though everyone else is calm and confident. The truth is that most of us feel fearful at least some of the time. We just don't like to show it. We believe that we must keep our feelings to ourselves because we are afraid of what other people are going to think of us. We are afraid of what they will say or do and that they will judge us harshly. Deep down, we are afraid that if other people knew how scared or worried we truly are, they would think we are weak or incompetent and, ultimately, unlovable.

It is this fear of not being loved that keeps the anxiety fires burning within us. While anxiety is triggered by stress, it is rooted in negative beliefs, such as the fear of being unlovable. We become anxious because we are afraid that whatever we fear will actually happen. To others, these fears may seem highly unlikely or even irrational, but for ourselves, the fears are real because they are based on ideas we believe to be true.

Difficult life events may be unavoidable, but we still have a choice about how to deal with those events. And developing personal traits such as strength and resilience, integrity, self-discipline, gratitude and compassion can help us to cope more effectively with life's trials. Facing life's challenges and struggling to overcome them can build these qualities over time, both consciously and unconsciously.

Past experiences

In their book, *Schema Therapy*, Eshkol Rafaeli, David P. Bernstein and Jeffrey Young describe psychological health as the ability to get one's needs met in an adaptive manner. Schemas are 'broad, pervasive themes regarding oneself and one's relationship with others, developed during childhood and elaborated throughout one's lifetime, and dysfunctional to a significant degree'. Schemas develop in childhood under the influence of a child's temperament and the child's damaging experiences with parents, siblings or peers.

Because they begin early in life, schemas become familiar and therefore comfortable, and so we try to hold on to them, even when they make us feel worse. We distort our view of the events and people in our lives in order to maintain the validity of our beliefs, focusing on the information that is consistent with our schema and ignoring that which is inconsistent. In other words, we interpret our lives not according to what is actually happening in the moment or who a person really is, but by what we believe subconsciously. Consequently, our interpretations often serve to reinforce these negative beliefs.

But these beliefs about ourselves and others and the ways we learn to cope with them can trigger feelings of anxiety and fear even in the most harmless situations. Here are just a few common but untrue beliefs we have about ourselves:

- I'm not good enough.
- I have to do for others, to be loved.
- I'm inadequate.
- I'm ugly.
- I'll never amount to anything.
- There's something wrong with me.
- I'm not worthy of love.
- Asking for help is a sign of weakness.
- I don't deserve to be happy.
- My thoughts and feelings don't matter.
- I have to make my parents proud of me.

According to Jerome Kagan, children who endured abuse or trauma or witnessed traumatic events are at higher risk of developing an anxiety disorder at some point in life. Whatever your genes or temperament, parenting practices will have a profound influence on whether you will ultimately become fearful and anxious later in life. Likewise, psych-iatrist Michael Liebowitz asserts that there is a connection between panic disorders and overprotective parenting. Trying to protect a sensitive child from harm might seem helpful, but it actually prevents the child from developing a natural and appropriate response to fear on his own. Consequently, these overexcitable children will tend towards anxiety as adults.

Some of the maladaptive methods people adopt to cope with their negative beliefs, difficult experiences and the painful feelings they create include surrender, overcompensation, defensiveness, depend-ence, entitlement, self-sacrifice and avoidance. In what Young terms the 'detached protector' mode, a person appears calm and in control, but it is an attempt to numb feelings and emotional needs and to dis-tance himself from fear, vulnerability and rejection.

However, these coping methods only create what psychologists call 'negative reinforcement', in which avoiding a feared situation only strengthens the behaviour. Avoidance provides temporary relief from unpleasant feelings, but this relief serves to reward the avoidant behaviour, reinforcing both the behaviour and the feelings of fear and anxiety associated with it.

We are often not even aware that we believe such things about our-selves or that we are coping in a negatively reinforcing way. As adults, these negative beliefs disguise themselves as thoughts or daydreams and show up in our lives as actions and reactions.

Penny is someone who knows what it's like to cope with fears. When-ever she had to make a presentation at work she would stop outside the meeting room and find her hands sweating and her mouth go dry and she'd begin to shake – all symptoms of anxiety. As she tried to calm herself down she would become increasingly nervous as she heard her own thoughts say, 'You're going to mess this up. Don't even bother. You never do anything right.' And then she grew even more nervous, so that when she did her presentation she did exactly what she believed about herself and she messed it up, thereby reinforcing the negative belief that she never does anything right and increasing her fear of pres-entations as well as her anxiety.

By becoming aware of her own negative beliefs, however, Penny came to realize that her anxiety about presentations was not due to her incompetence, but to her beliefs. One of them was that she never does anything right. The other was that if she fails, she will be rejected. So her anxiety was based on her fear of being rejected by people she admired, a belief that developed after disappointing her parents as a child.

While it is natural to want to do a good job and gain the respect of others, feeling like a failure and believing that you are not good enough if you don't get their respect is not healthy. The worst part about believing these kinds of negative ideas is the toll it takes on your self-esteem. The anxiety you feel is an unpleasant symptom. The belief that you will only be loved if you perform a certain way will crush your feelings of self-worth and your ability to live a happy life.

Unfortunately, we often grow up continuing to hang on to these beliefs because we are convinced that they are true. If your mother always told you that you were stupid or your father believed that you were a coward, it is difficult to think that there are any other ways of seeing yourself. You see yourself as your family saw you, because you trust them. In many cases, parents are trying to cope with their own negative beliefs about themselves, and the way they were treated when they were growing up, so they may not even be aware of the effect their words and actions have on their children or the negative beliefs they are creating.

Once Penny became aware of her fear of rejection she started to change the thoughts in her mind before presentations. Now, whenever she feels her hands begin to shake and her mouth go dry, she recognizes it as anxiety, caused by her fear of rejection. And then, instead of listening to the voice in her head that tells her she's going to mess it up, she pushes those thoughts aside and tells herself something else – she tells herself the truth. 'You are an intelligent, capable person who has worked hard and prepared well for this presentation. You will do a good job. And if anything goes wrong, it will be all right. You will not be rejected. You are not a failure. You can learn from your mistakes.' Armed with this new-found confidence and belief in herself as a person deserving of respect, Penny makes presentations that she is proud of. She still gets nervous sometimes, but she is learning to face her fears and not let the anxiety get the better of her.

Knowing that your parents are often struggling with their own faults and failings, and their own desires to be loved, without intending to hurt you, can help you to forgive them and to start taking responsibility for your own happiness. One of the most important things to remember about negative beliefs is that although you have held them for a long time, and you were probably told them by someone you trusted, they are not true. They were told to you by someone who did not know or see the real you. It isn't that person's fault and it isn't yours. But with some effort and awareness, and a mindful approach, you can begin to see yourself and treat yourself as you really are – a smart, strong, capable adult deserving of love. To learn what your own negative beliefs are, listen to your thoughts and your words. This will pull your beliefs out of your subconscious and into your conscious mind, where you can decide what to do with them rather than running on autopilot. And that is the first and best step towards alleviating fear. Face your feelings and your fears and accept them. And then start to let them go.

You may be struggling with fear because you have a predisposition for it. You may have a highly sensitive, creative personality or you may have an innate behavioural inhibition that has been part of your make-up since birth. You may also have learned some negative beliefs about yourself that you are still carrying with you. Although none of these factors will create a predestined life of anxiety, they will make you more likely to feel anxious in certain situations, and that can be challenging. Overcoming your fears is not easy. But by becoming aware of your environment, as well as yourself and your feelings, you can make the road a smoother one.

2

Where fear emerges

What are the situations that might create a feeling of fear? Once you can identify your own sources of fear, you can begin to work on dealing with them in a healthy way. If you are predisposed to feel fearful because of your genes, your temperament or your upbringing, certain situations can trigger fear for you whereas they may not for others. Many people experience a range of fears that can vary from mildly uncomfortable to debilitating. It's not important if other people find your fears unusual or strange or so common they are not worth mentioning. The key is to know what upsets you, because what upsets you matters. And when you know what upsets you, you can do something about it. In this chapter we'll discuss some common situations that can create fear. Think about whether any of these are true for you and then come up with a list of your own.

Learned fears

Some of the most common fears are situations, people or things that exist outside of our mind and outside of our comfort zone. Some of these include fear of flying, fear of heights, fear of the dark, and fear of failure. Many people are also afraid of spiders, snakes and dogs, while others are afraid of doctors, dentists, needles and germs. Fear of intimacy, fear of commitment and fear of abandonment are common fears that can cause significant relationship problems.

Through traumatic personal experiences or cultural influence, we have learned to become afraid of certain stimuli. Some of these fears are innate, and developed by nature to protect us from harm, such as a fear of wild animals, while others are cultural, such as a fear of an ambulance siren. Renowned child psychologist John Bowlby said that we can fear anything that we have learned can cause pain. Bowlby also noted that a fear of many cultural stimuli, such as the ambulance siren, could be hiding a natural fear, such as fear of death, in our subconscious attempts to make rational sense of them.

Fear, said Bowlby, can be aroused by natural situations that are not intrinsically harmless, such as sudden movement, darkness or separation from others. These conditions create an increased risk of danger, which we learn to fear. For example, a situation that triggers past memories of a frightening situation, such as visiting the site of a car accident, can create fear even though the site itself is no longer a source of danger.

Janet had always enjoyed football as a child, both playing in a team and attending local matches with her family. She was once at a football match with her parents and older sister when she was about ten years old. She went to get a soft drink by herself and when she came back to her seat the stadium was in chaos, with fans clambering over the fence to get onto the field and throwing punches at each other, while police with batons were shouting and trying to force everyone back. Hundreds of people were scrambling over the seats, desperately trying to get out. Janet struggled to fight her way through the mob, but she couldn't see her family anywhere. Eventually, a police officer took her to the police station, where they discovered that her family had all been injured in the fight and had been taken to hospital. She went to stay with her aunt until they had recovered. Janet is now 53 years old, and no longer goes to football matches. But when her husband watches it on television, just the sound of the cheering crowd can cause her mouth to go dry and her hands start shaking, often with tears in her eyes, and she has to leave the room.

Without becoming aware of these issues, however, these kinds of fears can easily turn into phobias, and begin to affect your normal routines and behaviour. Such fear is interpreted by the brain as a signal that danger is near, and so the body responds accordingly, with symptoms of anxiety.

As strange or irrational as they may seem to other people, none of these fears are wrong, as we fear the things we fear because of our own individual temperament and experiences. But that does not mean you have to live with it. Pretending you are not afraid when you actually are will only make the feared object or situation more powerful and you more afraid.

Unfamiliar situations

New experiences can be frightening because we do not always know what to expect. Whether you are moving to a new city, starting a new job or beginning the first day of school, you are entering unfamiliar territory.

According to what psychologists call 'the familiarity principle', we are attracted to what is familiar to us, simply because it is familiar. The more exposure we have to something or someone, the more highly we rate it. We recognize it, understand it and what is going to happen, and so we feel comforted and consequently seek more of those situations. Unfortunately, we are attracted to situations that are familiar whether they are good for us or not.

> Kelly grew up with an alcoholic father and vowed never to be in such a relationship when she grew up. But somehow she always found herself attached to alcoholics. She was subconsciously attracted to them because she recognized them. She knew they were not good for her, but they felt like home to her. And it was fear that stopped her from moving out of this comfort zone into unfamiliar territory, where she felt alone and scared at first, but truly happy and safe for the first time in her life.

Likewise, you can be attracted to familiar situations, such as the job where you are surrounded by old friends and familiar ways of doing things, but repelled by unfamiliar surroundings even if the new environment is a positive one.

> Stan had worked for the same company for ten years and he was bored. He wanted a promotion and he'd gone as far as he could go with his current employer. He needed a new challenge. But he felt comfortable where he was. He knew everyone in the office and he had made some good friends there. Everyone liked him and he had a core of buddies he went to lunch with every week and to the pub with on Friday nights. He wanted a new job, but the thought of leaving the familiarity of his friends and colleagues, as well as the respect he had worked so hard for over the years, kept him tied to his job and any chance of a move just a dream.

Social fears

Fear and anxiety can emerge when we encounter new people, either alone or in groups. You are at a party and someone introduces you to a group; suddenly you feel your cheeks burning, your mouth go dry and then you start to stutter. And it doesn't just happen at parties.

Melanie felt this kind of anxiety whenever she went to a shopping centre, the local park or even the school gates to pick up her kids. It wasn't the people themselves that she was afraid of but rather her fear of not fitting in, as well as her fear of saying the wrong thing. Melanie was shy and quiet and felt she was not very good at the kind of small talk that other parents often engaged in at the park. She knew she sounded awkward and so she came to fear these encounters so much that she began avoiding the other parents.

Public speaking is a kind of social fear but it's not just shy people who fear it. Many people fear facing an audience because they know they are being judged on their performance, their appearance, their thoughts and ideas and expression. You want to do a good job and you don't want to look or sound foolish. It's the fear not only of possible public humiliation but also social isolation that gets your heart thumping and your palms sweating.

Bowlby noted that social isolation, or loneliness, is one of the most profound and significant causes of fear. Humans are social animals and we have a deep need to feel that we belong and that we are accepted by our social group. Feeling isolated from others can make other fear-inducing conditions, such as unfamiliar places and sudden change, even more frightening.

Engaging with other people, however, is not always easy. There is the risk that you will say or do the wrong thing, or you could be anxious about opening up to others and exposing your vulnerabilities and fears to people who are not trustworthy. You can be afraid that you won't be able to hold up your end of the discussion in a one-to-one conversation and that you will bore the other person. Perhaps you feel overwhelmed by the banter of a big group or don't want to be the centre of attention. For some people, social situations can be so nerve-wracking that they fear their own physical response to their anxiety, and avoid situations that might cause them to blush, shake, sweat, speak with a croaking voice, vomit or need the bathroom.

Whether you are in a group or with one other person, and whether the situation is new or familiar to you, asserting yourself and your needs is an important skill. Fear can prevent you from telling someone at a party that the music is too loud or telling your husband that you need more help with the housework. Perhaps you fear their reaction or their opinion of you, or perhaps you avoid it because you don't think you deserve to get what you need. This kind of fear can also lead to finding yourself saying yes to things you don't want to do, like helping with a charity project when you are exhausted. Likewise, many people feel very uncomfortable giving and receiving compliments. Hearing something positive about yourself can make you feel like you don't deserve such attention and consequently question the other person's motives. Once again, it can often be your own thoughts and negative beliefs about yourself that stop you from having these conversations. But standing up for yourself and your needs is an essential part of developing a healthy self-esteem. Saying no to what feels wrong and yes to what feels right is not the same thing as being pushy or controlling, but it is a key to your personal happiness.

Many of the social fears we experience grow out of our own thoughts, which are created from the untrue beliefs we discussed earlier. If you believe you are going to fail at everything you attempt, that thought will run through your mind at every opportunity and will rise to the surface of your thoughts when you are at your most vulnerable, such as in a social situation. Most of the things we are afraid of happening, however, such as saying something so stupid that everyone will stop speaking to us, don't usually happen. Negative beliefs are not based on reality. But attempting social situations that make you feel afraid will help you to see what is real, and that you can meet new people, participate in discussions and feel relaxed around others.

Work worries

Work can often be the place where our fears emerge. Work creates a lot of stress for people and stress can trigger our fears, whether they involve anxiety over our performance or the fear that we are not making enough money. Demanding workloads, long hours, responsibilities, lack of job security, poor working environment and bullying at work are some of the common causes of work stress. According to a survey on anxiety in the workplace, 79 per cent of workers suffer from stress and anxiety every day.

A study in the journal *Occupational and Environmental Medicine* suggests that work is often a source of stress because stress arises from situations that are unpredictable, uncertain, ambiguous, involve conflict or include performance expectations. But developing personal coping skills, such as problem solving, time management, organization and assertiveness can help meet these pressures. Creating a healthy working environment through training, effective management practices and social support systems also help. Increasingly, employers are recognizing that they have a responsibility to help prevent and deal with stress among their employees.

Researchers have found that the sources of stress at work include those to do with the work itself and those associated with the context of work. The stress intrinsic to the job includes long hours, work overload, time pressure, difficult or complex tasks, lack of breaks, lack of variety and poor physical conditions, such as space, temperature and light. Being responsible for other people, as well as conflicting roles, can also cause stress. Having possibilities for advancement at work buffer against this stress, while underpromotion, lack of training and job insecurity increase it. Likewise, a good manager who promotes teamworking and a positive atmosphere can reduce stress levels, while a critical, demanding or unsupportive management style will build stress. Organizational change, such as restructuring, relocation or redundancies, especially when employees are not consulted, is another big source of stress. The lack of control over one's own work life is one of the key factors in the association between work and psychological ill health.

Workplace demands can also cause stress at home, as long and uncertain hours, job insecurity, relocation and work pressures take their toll on family responsibilities and family leisure time, a known stress reliever. Studies show that women are more likely to experience this kind of work/home stress because they are still responsible for more childcare and domestic chores than men. Women are also more likely to be in lower paid, lower status jobs and may additionally have to cope with sexual harassment and discrimination.

When a lack of control over one's working life is joined by high job demands, a lack of coping skills and low self-esteem, people can develop an increasing risk of experiencing stress. Individuals are not always in a position to change their working environment or company policies, but learning coping skills such as assertiveness, communication and time management can help. Still, these changes have limited effects unless the source of the stress is addressed. We'll discuss the importance of finding the work and the working environment that fit you in Chapter 12.

3

Triggers of anxiety and fear

Brian had had a long week. He was busy at work, his mother was sick and they were still unpacking from the house move a month ago. He didn't like coming home to a messy house. It made him angry. It wasn't just that he couldn't hang up his coat because the cupboard was full of boxes or that he had to step over the piles of kids' toys in the living room. There was something about clutter that made him feel really irritable. His wife worked full time too and he knew she was struggling to cope with the house and the kids. They'd already had one argument about it this week and he just couldn't face another one. He decided to have a drink to settle his nerves. But instead of calming him down, the whisky and soda seemed to ignite his anxiety, sending him into a tailspin.

Many of us can relate to Brian's dilemma. Our lives are often filled with pressures and deadlines and the stress of trying to manage many responsibilities, such as work and family. And those pressures can take a toll, leading us to feel a range of emotions, including anger, frustration and depression as well as anxiety and fear.

Certain situations can create an environment for fear to emerge, but there are also conditions that can trigger it. For example, coping with your in-laws' visit can be a situation that instils anxiety in some people, but when that situation is combined with triggers like a lack of sleep, the effect is like striking a match. Before you know it, your weekend with the family has turned into tears, arguments and everyone wondering what went wrong.

Studies have shown that people who experience frequent symptoms of fear or anxiety are also more likely to be in poor health. They are also more likely to smoke, drink and to be overweight. While scientists have not yet discovered whether fear causes poor health or poor health contributes to a fearful outlook, knowing that certain things can trigger feelings of fear can help you to take control. Poor diet, lack of sleep, stress, work, as well as the negative thoughts in your own mind can often turn an everyday situation into one in which you feel riddled with anxiety. Fortunately, these anxiety triggers are also parts of your life that you can change.

Diet

Caffeine, alcohol and sugar are three major stimulants that can trigger episodes of fear or anxiety. Many of us turn to a cup of coffee, a glass of wine or some chocolate when we begin to feel stressed or anxious because they are comforting and we believe they will help us relax.

However, caffeine is a stimulant, and whether it's coffee, tea or a soft drink it can make you feel jittery, shaky and edgy and can interfere with sleep. Alcohol can seem to take the edge off at first, but it doesn't last. As your body metabolizes the alcohol you can be left feeling edgy and depressed. Likewise, the initial spike in blood sugar level when you eat something sweet, the 'sugar rush', can feel like a relief but it soon wears off and can leave you feeling shaky, irritable and anxious.

Food sensitivities can also trigger irritability or other mood changes. Many people who experience fear and anxiety are sensitive, and that can include sensitivities to certain foods such as wheat, nuts, dairy, shellfish or gluten or to food additives. Exposure to foods to which you are sensitive can trigger not only a physical reaction, such as rashes or sneezing, but also symptoms of anxiety. If you think you may have a food sensitivity, see your doctor for an allergy test and try an elimination diet, where you stop eating anything you suspect is causing a reaction and take note of whether your symptoms disappear. You can often reintroduce the food gradually as your body develops a resistance to the allergen.

Certain medications also have negative side effects. Some drugs for the treatment of thyroid deficiency and asthma, as well as over-the-counter decongestants, cold remedies and weight loss supplements have been known to trigger symptoms of anxiety. Natural supplements have side effects too. St John's wort can lead to insomnia and green tea contains caffeine, a known anxiety trigger.

A thyroid problem has also been shown to cause anxiety symptoms in some people. Your thyroid is a gland in your neck that produces hormones which regulate your metabolism and energy levels. Too much of this hormone can make you feel nervous, irritable, sleepless and have heart palpitations. If you are experiencing symptoms of anxiety as well as a swelling in your neck, weight loss, weakness or fatigue, see your doctor.

Although there are no changes to your diet that will cure your fear, watching what you eat can help. Healthy eating will give you more energy, help you sleep better and provide a feeling of calmness. Here are a few tips:

Avoid foods that are fried, fatty, sugary and processed   They will tend to make you feel tired and add excess pounds.

Eat breakfast   Be sure to include some protein in your first meal, such as eggs, milk, yogurt, nuts or seeds, because protein will give you energy.

Include complex carbohydrates   These are foods such as wholewheat pasta and bread, brown rice and vegetables. Studies show that complex carbohydrates can increase the amount of serotonin in the brain, which has a calming effect.

Drink water   Your body needs water to function properly. Even mild dehydration can leave you tired and can affect your mood.

Eat lots of fruit and vegetables   Fresh foods contain lots of vitamins and minerals that are important for your physical and mental health.

Eat fish, walnuts and flaxseed   These foods contain omega-3 fatty acids, which not only lower cholesterol but also help the body to cope with stress by lowering blood pressure during stressful events.

Sleep

Getting enough sleep every night is essential to your health and to coping with fear and anxiety. When you don't get enough sleep you can feel irritable and tense, and feel the effects of stress much more acutely. If you are feeling fearful, a lack of sleep can make you feel worse. In addition, feeling anxious and fearful can make it difficult to fall asleep and stay asleep through the night. Studies show that people with chronic insomnia are at a high risk of developing an anxiety disorder. Because sleep and fear are so closely connected, it's essential to ensure that you are getting your forty winks every night.

According to the findings of a survey commissioned by the Anxiety Disorders Association of America, more than half of adults with a stress-induced sleep problem experience difficulty sleeping at least several times a week. Three-quarters of those adults say that their sleep problems have also increased their stress and anxiety. Eight out of ten adults have experienced some kind of sleep difficulty. Women are more likely than men to experience sleep problems, particularly feeling tired after sleep, and having difficulty falling asleep and staying asleep.

Sleeping recharges your brain and improves your focus, concentration and mood. If you are having trouble falling asleep or staying asleep, here are a few things you can do:

- Set aside 7–9 hours a night for uninterrupted sleep.
- Establish a calm bedtime routine, such as taking a bath, reading or listening to music before bed.
- Avoid watching TV or working on the computer before bed.
- Avoid caffeine and nicotine in the evening.
- Keep your bedroom cool, dark and quiet. Use blackout blinds or wear earplugs if necessary.
- Use your bedroom for sleeping and sex only. Don't watch TV in bed.
- Exercise regularly, but not less than 3 hours before bedtime.
- Get into bed only when you are tired. If you cannot sleep, get up and do something relaxing.
- If the problems persist, see your doctor.

Negative self-talk

Sometimes there is nothing in our environment to trigger feelings of anxiety but our own thoughts. And while they may be invisible to others, these thoughts are very real to us and create very real physical and emotional reactions.

As we discussed in Chapter 1, negative self-talk usually begins in childhood or with very early experiences where we believed the negative things that others told us. Negative self-talk is the thoughts we have in response to a situation that is familiar to us. For example, you can be preparing to go for a job interview, and your negative self-talk tells you that you are going to mess it up because you never do anything right. And then you feel your heart start to pound and your hands get sweaty. Or perhaps you are meeting a friend for coffee and you are going to a new place you have never been before. As you put on your coat, you think, What if I get lost? What if the bus is late? What if my friend doesn't show? These kinds of thoughts can not only give rise to anxiety symptoms, but stop you from living the life you want to live. The fear holds you back; you step away, hang up your coat and call your friend to cancel.

We can also put too much pressure on ourselves to act in a certain way once these negative thoughts take hold and we begin to feel their grip tightening on us. We don't want to appear in a bad light or upset anyone else, and so we try to force ourselves to act the 'right' way and the anxiety increases.

A lot of negative self-talk is based on low self-esteem. We continue to believe negative suggestions about ourselves because we have come to believe that they must be true. Thinking that you are not worthy enough or good enough or smart enough is easy to do when you have heard it often enough.

In his book *The Anxiety and Phobia Workbook*, Edmund J. Bourne explains that negative self-talk comes from your subconscious mind and so you often don't notice it's happening or the effect it's having on your mood, your feelings and your behaviour. But a single word or phrase or image can bring with it a flood of thoughts, memories and associations that can send you reeling into fear. It can be very difficult for others to understand what is going on or why you are afraid. Even when you try to explain it, your reasons seem irrational. But you continue to experience them and respond with fear because they sound and feel like the truth to you. Consequently, the negative self-talk leads you to avoid any situation that triggers those thoughts and feelings, creating a negative reinforcement of the situation and your fear.

Stress

Stress is the term used to describe the feelings that people experience when they struggle to cope with the demands made on them. These feelings are normal and affect everyone. Under stress, it is common to feel overwhelmed, tense or emotional.

Stress is caused when we are confronted with a threat to our safety. Your brain doesn't care whether it's an approaching tiger or an incoming email. It will react the same way, by tensing muscles and accelerating breathing and heart rate. Our body is preparing us to fight or run. This classic 'fight or flight' response is what creates the physical symptoms of fear and anxiety. We'll talk more about the way your body responds to stress and fear in Chapter 4.

Some stressors are external, like moving house, changing jobs or getting stuck in traffic. A new study in the journal *Nature* has revealed that being born and raised in a city is also a risk factor for anxiety and mood disorders. Furthermore, researchers at Brown University in the USA found that certain kinds of stressful life events cause panic symptoms to increase over time.

Other stressors are internal – the thoughts and feelings inside your mind that create uneasy feelings. These are the most common sources of stress, and include unrealistic expectations, uncertainties, apprehension and the way we feel about ourselves. We can also become stressed by too much information, boredom, isolation, time pressure, waiting and unpredictability. The degree to which you feel stressed by any of these conditions depends on your own temperament and experiences and your genes.

> Anne is an HSP, which means that she reacts much more strongly to sensory and emotional stimulation than other people. So while her colleagues are unfazed by the spreadsheets in the 2-hour meeting that has eaten into her lunch hour, Anne starts fidgeting, biting her nails and feeling sick after 40 minutes. Everyone thinks she's bored and inattentive, but she is feeling the effects of stress.

Stress is also one of the causes of a poor night's sleep, which in turn can trigger feelings of fear and anxiety. Stress does not cause anxiety or fear, but it can make them worse. Consequently, dealing with the stress in your life is essential.

Many environmental conditions can trigger fear and anxiety, especially in those who are highly sensitive. A change or uncomfortable levels of heat, cold, damp, noise, fresh air, smells, colours, textures and allergens can all become triggers.

According to Anxiety UK, if you answer yes to five or more of the following symptoms you may be suffering from stress, but it is important to seek guidance from your doctor:

- Obesity and overeating
- Increased or excessive drinking of alcohol
- Loss of appetite
- Increased smoking

- Increased coffee consumption
- Excessive and continuing irritability with other people
- Substance abuse
- Inability to make decisions
- Inability to concentrate
- Increased and suppressed anger
- Not being able to cope with life, feeling out of control
- Jumping from one job to another without finishing things
- Excessive emotion and crying at small irritations
- Lack of interest in anything other than work
- Permanently tired even after sleep
- Decreased sex drive/libido
- Nail biting.

One of the most common and difficult sources of stress is money. There never seems to be enough, and when we have it we want or need more. We argue with our loved ones over it. Stress usually builds during the winter months, thanks in part to the financial worries of increased heating bills and post-Christmas credit card debt. Try setting some savings aside every month in preparation for the festive season as well as birthdays and other special events, so you won't feel the pinch quite so hard when the bills come.

Becoming aware that certain factors are triggers for you can be enormously helpful, and mindfulness will allow you to be more aware of both your stress triggers and the ways they affect you, as well as providing a powerful means of letting those internal stressors go.

Learning to identify what makes you feel fearful and anxious, and the ways it affects you physically, emotionally and behaviourally, will help you to manage those feelings and the symptoms they cause. There are many triggers of fear and they are different for everyone. Brian finds an untidy house stressful, while it does not bother his wife. Likewise, Brian's anxiety is triggered by the alcohol he drinks to cope with the stress. The key is to discover what triggers fear and anxiety for *you*. Once you are aware of the triggers that cause your fear you will be able to manage your feelings, and your life, more effectively.

4

Paying attention when
your body speaks

Just as fear creates an emotional response in us, it can also create a physical response. And in the same way that we need to pay attention to the way that fear affects our feelings, it is important to become aware of the way it affects our bodies. One of the ways that mindfulness works is by making us more aware of the connection between mind and body. Your thoughts, feelings, beliefs and attitudes have an effect on your body. Feelings of stress and anxiety, for example, can make your hands sweat and your heart palpitate and, over time, raise your blood pressure. Likewise, the way we behave physically, such as what we eat and how much we exercise, affects our thoughts, moods and feelings as well.

Recognizing the signs of stress in your body means that you can change your thoughts and your focus to a more centred and relaxed mode, thereby reducing the stress as well as the physical symptoms, and improve your health and well-being.

Fear can cause a vast array of physical symptoms, such as a pounding heart and sweaty palms, but in the long term it can also contribute to significant health problems, like diabetes, heart disease, thyroid problems, asthma, allergies, chronic respiratory disorders, gastrointestinal conditions, eating disorders, sleep disorders and cancer. By listening to your body, however, and recognizing that pain, illness and discomfort can all be signs that your body, thoughts and emotions are in distress, you can help yourself to become healthier and happier in body, mind and spirit.

Pain, illness and the physical effects of fear

Constant worry, anxiety and fearful thoughts create stress, and your body responds to that stress in a way that can lead to health problems over time. Fear and worry trigger a fight or flight reaction in your body, which is an instinctive way of trying to cope with perceived danger by fighting it or running away. To prepare for either of these reactions, your body releases stress hormones, such as cortisol, to boost your blood sugar levels and blood fats (triglycerides) to give you energy. According to researchers, stress also stimulates the immune system in preparation for fighting infection and healing wounds, which causes inflammation in the body. Studies on stress have revealed that inflammation can contribute to a build-up of plaque that blocks the arteries, which can lead to heart problems. It also contributes to disorders caused by an imbalanced immune system, such as asthma.

In addition, the release of the hormone adrenaline creates an array of physical reactions such as dizziness, dry mouth, increased heart rate, nausea, headache, muscle tension, shortness of breath, sweating and trembling. Most of us are familiar with these symptoms, as they occur whenever we feel afraid or anxious. It's the body's way of preparing us for action.

One of the most common chronic conditions connected to stress is allergies. Studies have shown that even small amounts of stress, anxiety and fear can make your allergic reactions not only more severe, but last longer. In a laboratory experiment, researchers at Ohio State University found that the allergic skin reactions of participants who were moderately anxious were 75 per cent larger than the same person's reaction when they were not anxious. Furthermore, the more fearful and anxious the participant, the greater their allergic reaction. These highly anxious people were also four times more likely to have a stronger reaction even a day after the stressful event, causing researchers to surmise that stress can cause a strengthening of the allergic reaction, even to substances that the subject was not previously allergic to. Such delayed allergic reactions, according to scientists, typically do not respond to common allergy treatments such as antihistamines.

The trouble is that the brain doesn't know the difference between the fear of an oncoming tiger and the fear of rejection on a first date, and so all that energy and all those stress hormones, instead of being released through physical activity, remain in the body and create harmful conditions such as immune system suppression, digestive disorders, blood sugar disorders and heart problems. While stress caused by worry and fear can cause illness, having a serious health condition can also cause significant worry and fear, perpetuating the cycle of fear and illness.

Janet had felt unhealthy all her life. She knew she needed to improve her diet, which consisted of too much junk food, especially when she was feeling afraid or worried. Over the years she had gained weight and developed diabetes. While diets helped her to lose a little bit of weight, she always gained it back and now her doctor was suggesting that she might need medication to control her blood sugar, as well as medication for her anxiety. Janet didn't want to depend on drugs, so she decided that whenever she felt upset, she would just tell herself to stop worrying about it.

But trying to hold in negative emotions does not help. Whatever we are feeling will manifest itself in some way, either through emotional expression, such as crying or talking, or through the body, where the stress response creates pain, illness, inflammation and can lead to chronic health conditions. Suppressing emotions also uses up vital energy and nutrients that we need to support our bodily functions, and we can consequently become drained, fatigued and weakened by the effort. Our emotional health is also affected by suppressing our feelings as it can lead to frustration, anger, depression, low self-esteem and self-criticism, all of which create their own painful physical symptoms.

According to Dr Arthur Janov, author of *Why You Get Sick, How You Get Well*, emotional pain is created when a child lacks love and nurturing. If this pain is not addressed, it will cause physical and emotional illness later in life. The energy from painful feelings is bottled up, the pressure builds and chronic health problems often develop. Unfortunately, many people have learned to ignore or avoid facing their feelings because they are so painful. But ignoring them doesn't make them go away. In many cases, those feelings only dig deeper into your physical well-being and create cell damage, as well as exhaustion due to the energy needed to keep the pain at bay, which in turn can leave you susceptible to depression and anxiety. Repression, or holding your feelings in, Janov says, is the foundation of many diseases, both emotional and physical. Instead of treating the symptoms of this kind of illness with medication, for example, it's far more effective to treat the cause of the sickness and address the emotional need at the root of the problem. Furthermore, you need to do more than simply understand your emotions. You need to feel them. According to Janov's studies, when adults deal with their unfulfilled need to be loved, their stress hormone levels drop and their immune system improves.

Part of what makes addressing our emotional needs so difficult is the deep-rooted fear that, since no one gave you what you needed, you are alone and there is no one there to help. The benefit of becoming an adult, however, means that you are not alone. You can reach out for help from others. And you can help yourself.

Since burying her feelings was only making her feel worse, both emotionally and physically, Janet decided to get professional help. She discovered the root of her illness was fear, beginning with her fear of losing her parents, a fear that she had carried around with her all her life. Once she let those feelings out, through talking and journalling and became more aware of her fears and how they affected her, she began to gain control of her eating habits, and her health began to improve. She stopped trying to suppress her feelings by eating and instead faced her fears. Using mindfulness techniques, she learned to express her feelings purposefully and mindfully, rather than unconsciously trying to keep them at bay. Instead of letting worries, negative thoughts about herself and food temptations fill her day, she learned to focus on the present moment and find the joy that was all around her.

Sensitive people's physical response to stress

Everyone responds to long-term stress and emotion in different ways, and sensitive people are particularly prone to the physical as well as the emotional repercussions of fear. Because they absorb so much sensory and emotional information from the world around them, sensitive people can easily become overstimulated and overwhelmed, which stresses both their mind and their body and ultimately creates pain, fatigue, insomnia and digestive or immune problems as well as a variety of symptoms. Sensitive people also tend to develop allergies and sensitivities to certain foods and environmental and chemical agents. They are vulnerable to blood sugar disorders, migraines and headaches, fibromyalgia and chronic fatigue, intense premenstrual syndrome symptoms, skin problems such as eczema or cold sores, as well as asthma, colds, flu and infections.

For highly sensitive types, stress can easily become overwhelming because of the volume of information they absorb. They also absorb the emotions of others, which the average person is better able to block out. So spending time around negative or angry people or conflicts, for example, can create serious health problems as well as emotional distress and exhaustion for the HSP. Likewise, sensitive people can become stressed by seemingly harmless everyday places and activities like parties, supermarkets, meetings, TV violence, public transport, unfamiliar environments, noise and crowds.

In an attempt to cope with sensory and emotional overload, the HSP will often become anxious, nervous, upset, impatient, irritable or withdrawn. For sensitive types, becoming aware of the conditions that trigger overwhelming feelings for you is the key to keeping your mind calm and your body well.

Body language

Our body responds physically to the levels of stress we subject it to. We tend to deal with pain, illness and physical problems by treating the symptoms instead of the root problem, and see those symptoms as a source of irritation. But in the same way that our feelings are trying to point us to the cause of our emotional pain, our body can also alert us to the root of our problems by forcing us to stop our mindless habits and become aware of our physical needs. In this way the body is crying out for help, and by listening closely we can hear what it is trying to tell us. For example, digestive problems often occur when we cannot stomach a situation or we develop foot ailments when we are afraid to take the next step.

According to author Louise Hay and scientist Bruce Lipton, your thoughts and feelings not only affect your health and well-being but your body reveals your subconscious beliefs and your true feelings through physical symptoms. This awareness of how the body responds to your emotional state means that struggling to manage what is going on in your heart or your mind or your life, for example, can cause digestive problems. Likewise, feelings like resentment and bitterness can cause pain and inflammation and an inflexible attitude can create stiff joints. Repressed hurt feelings can present themselves as arthritis, while deep hatred, guilt or grief can eat away at you like cancer. Back pain may be an indication of feeling a lack of emotional support. Negative feelings such as shame, guilt, fear, anxiety, anger and hate will weaken your body, while positive emotions such as joy, love, understanding, forgiveness, acceptance and trust will strengthen it. Studies also show that depression, for example, creates a greater risk of heart disease than hypertension or obesity because depressed people have given up hope.

Here are some physical symptoms that we have all experienced and the associated emotional and mental states that trigger them:

Headaches   A 'knock on the head' indicating that you are ignoring your own needs.

Eye problems   You are not seeing something clearly.

Hearing problems   You may be tuning out what you don't want to hear.

Neck and shoulders   Your neck is the bridge between your mind and your body and stiffness here can indicate a conflict between emotional and material needs.

Arms and hands   You need them to reach out to others for help. Are you holding back?

Lung and heart problems   Feeling unloved and not loving others. Fear restricts and makes you breathe shallowly and makes your heart pound. Express your love, so that your own heart is full and you can breathe deeply. Most importantly, show love for yourself and feel the love that you have inside you. Expressing love will attract love from others.

Spine and back   Your spine supports you, so back pain indicates a feeling of lack of support and challenges in life that you are struggling to cope with. Middle and lower back pain suggest you are burdened by hurt from the past or childhood issues, leaving you feeling insecure and anxious.

Liver problems   Negative emotions such as resentment and anger can weaken your liver.

Infertility   Reproductive problems suggest feelings of insecurity, that the world is not a safe place. Repressing your creativity can also lead to problems in this area.

Hips and legs   The bottom half of your body often reflects deep trauma, jealousy and emotional pain, causing soreness and an inability to move forward in life and a sense of lack of support.

Knees and feet   Negative emotions, such as hurt, tend to fall to the lowest part of your body and often reflect long-held painful feelings from childhood that keep us from taking a step forward.

Because physical symptoms appear as the body's cry for help, the emotional cause of those symptoms may have happened a long time ago. It's the long-term toll that negative or repressed feelings take on the mind and the body that creates damage. If you felt unloved growing up, you may only be experiencing the effects of that pain as an adult, as a heart condition or back pain. And while you may have found a loving relationship now, the relaxation and happiness you feel can trigger the release of those old negative feelings because your subconscious mind and your body feel that it's safe to let them out. We often blame our current partner for the feelings that arise, but it's often the pain of the past that we are really experiencing. The key is to deal with your own feelings and not to point the finger at someone else or to bury those feelings any longer.

The important thing to recognize is that your mind and your body work together and affect each other, so that when you experience physical symptoms of any kind, they are an indication that your thoughts and feelings are experiencing the same kind of pain. Ignoring your body's attempts to communicate with you will only exacerbate your health problems as well as your emotional issues. You can begin to heal your body by looking at the feelings that caused the pain or the illness. By expressing those feelings and releasing that negativity you can heal your mind, your body and your heart.

5

Discover who you really are

Knowing who you are and what you need is essential to overcoming fear. Without a clear understanding of the kind of person you are and your needs, fear can easily take over, filling in the gaps in your self-esteem with self-doubt and preventing you from fulfilling your potential. Everyone has a purpose in life, and fear can prevent you from finding out what that purpose is as well as stopping you from reaching it.

Jane had always worked hard at her job, but she knew deep down it wasn't fulfilling. She often came home feeling exhausted and bored and dreading Mondays. She worked as an administrative assistant for a big construction company and for years she had drifted from job to job in the hopes of finding something better. Whenever she felt that familiar bored and exhausted feeling, she put it down to an overbearing boss or long working hours and handed in her notice. But the change from one company to another never made much difference. Even with a great boss, she still felt anxious and depressed. She knew she needed to do something different, but she just didn't know what it was or how to find it. Worst of all, when friends asked her what she liked to do, she had no idea. She had spent her life doing what other people liked to do and what she thought she *should* do and so her understanding of who she really was and what she really needed to find fulfilment remained buried and out of sight.

Jane began reading books and spending some time thinking about what she liked to do and the way that certain activities made her feel. She noticed that she often felt irritable after spending time on tasks that required a lot of close attention to detail and after being around large groups of people. Conversely, she discovered that taking a few hours to do something by herself, such as read or bake or garden, seemed to recharge her batteries. She also found that when she had spent time alone she felt calmer, more relaxed and more energized, which led to her rediscovering a passion for drawing that she thought she had simply outgrown.

Learning more about herself and paying attention to the way she felt when she engaged in certain activities meant that not only Jane could take control of her life and reduce her anxiety but also build her self-confidence. She knew what worked for her and what didn't, and while it was a challenge to assert her needs to others, with practice and her developing self-esteem, she began to feel less afraid of what others might think of her. She also became less afraid of stepping out into the world, because she knew how to take care of herself. Sometimes she had to make the difficult choice to say no to friends' invitations to parties because she knew she would feel overwhelmed by the number of people and the noise. But making choices that restored her sense of peace and refuelled her energy reserves made Jane feel good about her decisions. She began to look at different options for work, and explored the possibilities for a career change. In the meantime, she took the time she needed to relax and do things she enjoyed doing, even when some of her friends thought she was wasting her time or accused her of being unsociable. She knew it was right for her and she felt happier as a result. And the friends that understood her needs were the ones who stayed friends, enjoying both her company when she did socialize, and her new-found sense of joy.

Knowing yourself well means that you can take control of your own life and find ways to get what you need, whether it's more friends, deeper relationships or more time to yourself. Once you start giving yourself what you need, you will feel calmer, happier and more confident because you will no longer be yearning for what you need or depending on anyone else to give it to you. You will no longer be willing to accept alternatives that don't suit you. Recognizing that you can say yes to what feels right and no to what feels wrong for you personally, regardless of what is right or wrong for other people, is one of the most empowering things you can do. And soon you will be filling up the dark spaces in your life with love and self-assurance, leaving no more room for fear.

How to build self-understanding

So how do you start to learn about who you are? Often, it's this first step that prevents us from unravelling the mystery of our undiscovered selves. And in order to change something in your life, you need not only the willingness to change but you also need new information. Without it, you will keep repeating the same habits and behaviours and patterns simply because you don't know what else to do. To find a way out of the fog created by lack of understanding, you need to know there are alternative paths.

Psychologist Carl Jung wrote the book *Psychological Types*, in which he stated that understanding one's own personality type is crucial because, as he wrote, 'it is one's psychological type which from the outset determines and limits a person's judgment'. Knowing what type of person you are can give you access to your own needs and allow those judgements to be based on clarity and understanding.

Jung's theory of personality categorized people into types of psychological function. These functions are thinking, feeling, sensing and intuition, and personality can be described as a combination of these functions. Jung also proposed that these functions are expressed as either introversion or extroversion.

Extroversion means 'outward-turning' and refers to a preference for drawing energy from the external world of action, people and things. Extroverts gain energy from being out in the world and feel drained spending time alone and in reflection. Introversion means 'inward-turning' and these kinds of people are energized by the internal world of thoughts, ideas and reflection. To recharge their energy, introverts need quiet, solitary time away from activity and other people.

Because they need time alone and can feel easily overwhelmed and stressed around other people, introverts seem to be more likely to become anxious and fearful. Several studies have found a close correlation between introversion and fearfulness. In one study, researchers suggested that introverts have greater self-awareness than extroverts and that those who have high self-awareness are often more anxious in social situations. Another study found that introverts struggle with social relationships because of their fear of being negatively judged by others. Likewise, introverts often doubt that they have the ability to make successful impressions on others and so their social interactions are often hindered by their fears.

Discovering that you are an introvert, however, does not mean that you are doomed to a life of fear, anxiety and social failure. It simply means that you have different needs from someone who is an extrovert and that by taking care of yourself and your needs you can feel more relaxed and more confident.

The Myers–Briggs Type Indicator and the Keirsey Temperament Sorter are personality-type tests based on Jung's theories of psychological type. Isabel Briggs Myers and Peter B. Myers' book *Gifts Differing* and David Keirsey's book *Please Understand Me II* provide a wealth of information on personality types, including temperament, character and intelligence.

Keirsey has developed the concept of four major types of temperament, which he calls Idealist, Rational, Artisan and Guardian. Artisans, for example, talk mostly about what they see right in front of them, about what they can get their hands on, and they will do whatever works, whatever gives them a quick, effective payoff, even if they have to bend the rules. Idealists, on the other hand, speak mostly of what they hope for and imagine might be possible for people, and they want to act in good conscience, always trying to reach their goals without compromising their personal code of ethics.

> Katherine had always been teased in school for being a cry-baby and criticized as an adult for being too shy, too quiet and too sensitive. She wanted to be like everyone else, but she couldn't help getting emotional at sad movies and even crying over tragic events she heard on the news. While she struggled to overcome what she and others saw as her 'flaws', she grew increasingly anxious and insecure, with the belief that she just wasn't good enough and that perhaps there was something wrong with her. It was only when her sister invited her along to the centre for elderly people where she volunteered that Katherine found a place where her warmth and sensitivity to others' feelings were not a detriment but a welcome asset. She found it not only easy to listen to people but she also enjoyed it, and she noticed how good it made her feel to be helping others. She didn't have to try to be like anyone else. All she had to do was be herself and suddenly her natural sense of compassion and empathy was improving the lives of people around her, as well as building her own self-esteem. She wasn't flawed at all, she realized. She was simply meant for something special.

While you are reading and learning all this new information about yourself, it may be a good idea to keep a journal of what you have discovered. Additionally, writing in a journal can be an effective way of releasing stress as well as providing an opportunity for expressing your thoughts, feelings and fears. Writing can often be an appealing outlet for introverts in particular, since it's a quiet, solitary pursuit that allows you to express your creativity. And getting your thoughts and fears on paper can help to limit their power over you.

Keeping a journal can also help you to see patterns in your own behaviour and to recognize your values, tastes, interests and beliefs. You may think, for example, that you enjoy sport because your family always has and you grew up with it. But writing in a journal can reveal otherwise. You may notice that you write how much you dread going swimming and that you keep coming up with excuses to miss games with your friends. These kinds of things are not always clear when you are holding fast to a belief about yourself you have had for a long time. But writing is often a doorway to your subconscious mind, the part of your thinking that drives your behaviour but that you are not aware of. You may think you love sport or parties or watching a particular TV programme, but in fact you may be engaging in any number of activities and/or behaviours because of deep-rooted beliefs that may not even be yours. Journalling can help bring these subconscious beliefs to the surface. We'll talk more about the benefits of keeping a journal in Chapter 10.

Sometimes it can also be helpful to ask other people what we are really like. After all, your friends and family have a different perspective on your behaviour and your personality than you do. Katherine's mother, for example, could see that her daughter had a keen interest in helping others because she was always talking about other people's feelings. She also saw how excited Katherine became when she talked about the importance of helping others. Katherine assumed that everyone thought this was important and so she did not think it was a special trait. But after talking to her mother she realized that this was something she was particularly interested in and an area in which she had a natural ability.

It takes courage to talk to others and to hear the truth. And of course other people's opinions can come with their own agendas and biases. But asking questions about ourselves with those close to us is well worth the effort and the risk. If you ask enough people, you will see patterns emerge or similar kinds of comments repeated. Jane, for example, decided to ask her friends what they thought her real passions were, and again and again her friends described her as a very creative, artistic person, although Jane had never thought of herself that way.

The benefits of a fearful, anxious temperament

Personality traits such as introversion and sensitivity can make people more likely to experience fear and anxiety. However, they also tend to have many positive qualities, including creativity, compassion and even giftedness.

Many sensitive or gifted individuals also hold high standards for themselves and possess an acute awareness of complexities and consequences. They also have a strong desire for self-determination and self-actualization, which helps in the understanding of themselves, their needs and their potential.

Part of what causes anxiety is the intensity of emotions and energy absorbed from others and from the drive to be creative. So doing something creative helps to channel that energy and release the negative feelings. The drive to do something meaningful also creates energy, and that persistence needs an outlet. Find what you are passionate about and do it. You will not only feel happier but also more relaxed.

A recent study has also suggested that people who are anxious are more likely to be persistent, a personality trait that allows you to be persevering, ambitious, conscientious and perfectionist, and you consequently get more done and achieve more on your own. You also tend to work harder because you cannot tolerate procrastination or the fear of deadlines. It's a type of motivation that allows you to get things done.

Many people who are fearful or anxious are also highly sensitive, which means they have a more sensitive nervous system and absorb and process sensory information more intensely. One research study found that people who have an exaggerated 'startle' reflex may find it harder to regulate emotional arousal, which suggests that sensitive types are often overstimulated and can easily feel anxious as a result.

According to Dr Elaine Aron, author of *The Highly Sensitive Person*, there are many benefits to being the highly sensitive type. First, you have a keen awareness of your environment, so that you know what is going on around you and you are highly intuitive. Sensitive people are also usually creative. According to Aron:

> Creativity by definition involves putting together things that are not usually thought of as belonging together, and that requires a deeper and fuller processing of experiences, situations, and possibilities. (This is an especially valuable trait in the workplace.)

Many people are not aware that they are creative, however, because of a lack of confidence or because of experiences with criticism that led to the repression of their creative expression.

Compassion and empathy are also common in sensitive, creative, anxious types. They tend to have a high awareness of their own feelings as well as those of other people, and can imagine what those feelings must be like and so express sympathy and concern. All kinds of communication skills seem to be a strength as well. Being aware of subtleties in the environment and in others means you are able to pick up non-verbal cues to people's needs and emotions.

Since sensitive people are more emotional, they can sense the full emotional and intellectual consequences as well as experience all emotions more intensely, including love, hope, joy, pride and awe.

Aron suggests that HSPs belong to the 'priestly advisor' class, in that their awareness of their environment and the people around them enable them to possess information that others do not have access to. In this way, sensitive people are typically consultants, counsellors, historians, scientists, artists and healers. The world needs them to help them make informed decisions that take all consequences into consideration, as well as to use their natural concern for social justice. Sensitive, anxious people are often gentle people who dislike discord, anger and violence and will seek to encourage peace wherever they go, both for their own peace of mind and for the sake of others.

James Kagan has studied anxious, sensitive or what he calls 'high-reactive' people extensively, and found that those who learn to adapt to their trait tend to have support either from one or two friends or from finding something they are good at which boosts their confidence. Other adaptive qualities of an anxious temperament include caution, introspection and the ability to work alone and to be self-motivated. They also tend to avoid danger because they are typically more restrained. They are generally conscientious, careful and well prepared, as well as hard-working people.

The important thing to remember, and the thing that has helped Jane and Katherine to overcome their fear and feelings of anxiety, is to tell yourself that no matter what happens, you will be okay. Even if your fears do come true and you lose your job or your wife leaves you, you will still be okay. And that's because you know who you are and what you need and you are able to give yourself what you need, so what other people do doesn't matter that much. Fear often arises from the belief that something bad is going to happen and that you won't be able to cope if it does. But once you know who you are, you will know that you have resources you can rely on right inside you, all the time.

Perhaps you have discovered that you are an HSP and also very creative, so that when stressful events occur, you know you can lean on your creative outlet and feel better. Perhaps, like Katherine, you have found that you are not a weakling, like the boys at school teased you about being, but in fact you are a compassionate, caring person and you are now able to use those abilities as strengths. She is now working as a professional counsellor and she feels more confident than ever because she is doing what feels right for her as well as benefiting from the pleasure of helping others.

Giving yourself what you need and doing what you feel passionate about will fill you up in a way that nothing else can, providing you with the confidence and strength to weather life's storms. Jane and Katherine have learned more about themselves and what they each need as individuals, and so while they are prone to experiencing anxiety, they know they will be all right. You will be all right too, because you have the one thing that you need to get through anything – you have you, and that's something you can always count on.

Part 2

THE MINDFUL WAY

6

How mindfulness works

Mindfulness is never about doing something perfectly, because it is not about doing or accomplishing at all. It is about allowing things to be as they are, resting in awareness, and then, taking appropriate action when called for. Silence, deep listening, and non-doing are often very appropriate responses in particularly trying moments — not a turning away at all, but an opening toward things with clarity and good will, even toward ourselves. Out of that awareness, trustworthy skilful responses and actions can arise naturally, and surprise us with their creativity.

(Jon Kabat-Zinn)

Mindfulness is a way of developing awareness and paying attention to the present moment. Using techniques like meditation, breathing and yoga, we can become more aware of the thoughts that can lead us to feelings of fear and anxiety. Because sensitive, anxious people often feel overwhelmed by their emotions and their surroundings, mindfulness can be an effective way of managing those feelings and our response to our environment.

Professor Mark Williams of Oxford University describes mindfulness as doing things knowing that you are doing them. Mindfulness enables people to find stillness in the middle of a frantic world. When you are stressed, your attention and concentration fade and you begin to panic. Mindfulness helps you to regain a sense of calm.

According to a Mental Health Foundation survey in 2010, 86 per cent of people believe that 'people would be much happier and healthier if they knew how to slow down and live in the moment'. Learning how to slow down in the face of a busy work life, child care, commuting and money worries can be difficult. But mindfulness isn't necessarily something to add to your to-do list as much as a different way of experiencing your world.

Based on ancient Zen Buddhist techniques, mindfulness has evolved from a religious practice to a tool that anyone can use, helping you to reduce stress, calm your emotions and even relieve pain and illness. Mindfulness techniques have even been used in the treatment of depression, anxiety disorders, substance abuse and other health conditions.

Mindfulness is not a religious experience, however, or at least it doesn't have to be. You don't have to fast or go on a retreat in the woods for 10 days or wear clothes made out of bamboo. Mindfulness is an attitude, a way of seeing the world and your place in it in a way that makes you feel calm and grounded instead of harassed and harried. Anyone can bring mindfulness into their lives and feel the benefits of it. For those who are particularly vulnerable to stress, anxiety and fear-based feelings, mindfulness can be the key to living the life you really want.

> Rebecca had always wanted children. She grew up dreaming of the day when she would be the mother of a large family. But when she got married, she discovered that she wasn't able to have children for medical reasons. Heart-broken, she condemned the tragedy of her life as unfair and cruel, and felt that she was simply a helpless victim. She grew angry, depressed and her self-esteem crumbled. Her husband couldn't stand her despair and eventually they divorced. A few years later, Rebecca had rebuilt her life, finding a new job in a new town that she loved. She had learned some mindfulness techniques, such as yoga and meditation, as a way of relaxing and dealing with her fears, and she became more comfortable with her life. It was then that she met David, a single father of three children. When David introduced Rebecca to the children, she felt like she had come home. She and David married and she found herself the mother of a loving family. It hadn't happened the way she'd expected or planned, but she couldn't imagine being happier. She had learned to accept events in her life and enjoy it as she focused on the joy of each moment, rather than worrying about the future or feeling angry at the past.

Here are some of the main elements of the mindful way of living:

Live in the moment   Stress and anxiety and the negative feelings that come with them are usually caused by our own thoughts. We worry about something that's happened in the past or fear the consequences of an event in the future. By focusing on today, right now, you can let go of trying to control the past or the future and relax into appreciating whatever is happening now. Children often live in the moment. When they play, they are not thinking of what time it is or what they have to do later. They become absorbed in what they are doing and allow events to unfold naturally, and consequently their enjoyment of their experiences is palpable. A childlike enthusiasm can exist in adults too when we allow ourselves to enjoy and appreciate the world in front of us.

Awareness While being aware of what is happening around you in the present moment, become aware of the way you feel in the moment. What are your thoughts now? What are you feeling as you experience the world? How is your body responding to your environment? Become aware of your breathing. Awareness of your feelings and moods allows you to become more in tune with your own experiences as well as how you affect others and how they affect you. Paying attention to your own responses is key to learning how to manage your emotions and bring more joy into your life by allowing you to shift from autopilot to noticing the life you are living right now.

Open to experience Avoiding situations, people, thoughts or feelings that seem fearful to you is often an instinctive way of coping, but it can be painful in the long term. Avoiding things does not make them go away. Face your thoughts, feelings and experiences openly, knowing that these sensations can make you more aware of yourself and your needs. Step back and look at your own thoughts, feelings and difficulties in life objectively, so that you can see things for what they are with clarity and openness and a non-judgemental attitude. Let go of your attachment to certain outcomes, such as the idea that you won't be happy until you get a certain job or marry a certain kind of man. Letting go of a specific path allows your mind to open to possibility and generates the creativity and ideas that can ultimately lead you in the right direction for you, without the confusion of 'should' and 'ought to' getting in the way.

Acceptance Trying to control anything or anyone will only lead to frustration and anxiety, as well as wear away your self-esteem. So too will feeling like a victim. Instead of trying to force your will on others or change your circumstances, accept that you are where you are in the moment and in your life for a reason. There is no good or bad. They just are what they are and you do not need to feel bad about yourself for your circumstances or your negative feelings. Accepting them, while uncomfortable or frightening, is liberating. They no longer have control over you when you face them. Things change and you cannot predict what will happen or how. But you can stay true to your own purpose and your own values, despite life's changing seasons. Accept that other people have to learn on their own as well. Other people have their own selves to understand in their own way, so do not judge them as they are struggling to climb their own mountains. In *Mindfulness in Plain English*, author B. H. Gunaratana explains, 'Mindfulness is objective, but it is not cold or unfeeling. It is the wakeful experience of life, an alert participation in the ongoing process of living.'

Compassion   Becoming aware of your own feelings will open you up to the feelings of others, and to your sense of empathy and compassion, both for other people and for yourself. It's important to be gentle with yourself. Listen, and be there for others, not for what they can do for you or because they will appreciate you, but because they need you to care. And the feeling of connection that mutual compassion nurtures will liberate you from any restraint you may have placed on yourself. Love, compassion and understanding are not a sacrifice – they are the free-flowing effects of an open heart and a strength of character.

The mind–body connection

Mind–body specialist Dr James Gordon says that the mind and body are essentially inseparable:

> The brain and peripheral nervous system, the endocrine and immune systems, and indeed, all the organs of our body and all the emotional responses we have, share a common chemical language and are constantly communicating with one another.

Mindfulness practice includes techniques that enhance the mind–body connection and encourage the mind's positive impact on the body. These techniques include meditation, prayer, art, music, dance, yoga, t'ai chi, qigong, and deep breathing.

Deep breathing is a mind–body mindfulness practice that increases the mind–body connection. Breathing mindfully makes an enormous difference to your mental and physical health because your entire body, including your brain, needs oxygen to function properly. When you are stressed, depressed or anxious the body's supply of oxygen is depleted because we tend to breathe shallowly, our posture is poor and the lungs don't get enough oxygen.

Meditation and mindfulness master Thich Nhat Hanh explains, 'When your mind is there with your body, you are established in the present moment. Then you can recognize the many conditions of happiness that are in you and around you, and happiness just comes naturally.'

How mindfulness works in the brain

The brain is divided into two hemispheres. The left is associated with analytical thinking, logic and rational processing. The right brain is involved in abstract thought, visual and spatial perception, creativity and emotional expression. According to neuroscientist Dr Shanida Nataraja, left-brain thinking dominates the behaviour of most people in the Western world, which results in too much thinking, too much worrying and a frantic way of living. Mindfulness can not only calm the anxiety of daily life but also help us shift from left-brain to right-brain thinking. When we make this shift, we become more relaxed, more creative and better able to see the possibilities.

Many people believe they are not the creative type, but everyone has the potential to be creative. It is simply a matter of turning off the logical mind and engaging the creative mind. You cannot be creative if you are running from one activity or one thought to the next. This kind of left-brain activity stimulates the sympathetic nervous system, releasing adrenaline in the fight or flight response that creates feelings of stress. The right brain operates under the parasympathetic nervous system, which restores the body to equilibrium, allowing it to relax and recuperate from stress. In this right-brain state, you are relaxed enough to see the possibilities and options in life, and this is where creativity emerges. No matter what kind of person you are, a relaxed mind is a creative mind.

In a 2007 study at the University of Toronto, scientists determined that people have two distinct ways of experiencing the world. The default network becomes active when not much else is happening and you begin to think, about yourself and other people, about plans and problems and things you have to do, about the past and the future, while essentially ignoring the world around you. Researchers called this network the 'narrative' because you are creating stories of your experiences.

The other way of experiencing life is called 'direct experience', in which different areas of the brain are active. This kind of thinking involves the perception of sensory information, such as sights, sounds, smells, tastes and touch. In this way, you stop thinking about the past or future, and you pay attention instead to the warmth of the sun on your face or the scent of the lilac bushes as you walk down the street. You don't notice these sensory details, however, when you are in narrative mode, because your brain is absorbed in thinking.

Narrative thinking is essential for planning, goal setting and organizing, while direct experience allows you to become aware of information in your world more clearly and accurately in real time, rather than imagining past or future events. You experience life as it happens, releasing you from the confines of your past and your expectations of the future. In an experiment, people who practised mindful meditation regularly were able to differentiate between these two modes and could choose which experience they wanted. People who did not practise mindful awareness tended to automatically take the narrative path.

People who are susceptible to fear and anxiety, such as HSPs, are naturally more aware of the sensory information in their environment. They are in direct experience mode all the time, highly aware of the sights, sounds and smells and feelings of other people around them, as well as the effect that sensory information has on themselves, both physically and emotionally. The difficulty for this type of person comes when they become overwhelmed by such sensory information, which can happen when they are in a too crowded or too noisy environment, for example, and the person often responds with feelings of fear, stress, anxiety or depression.

For a sensitive person, the level of sensory information they absorb is much higher than for other people, and so they need to take care of themselves and engage the parasympathetic nervous system in a way that works for them. They may need more time alone, more sleep, more quiet time in nature than the average person, in order to release themselves from the stress of overstimulation and regain the state of calm, creative relaxation. When they can find the environment that works for them, sensitive and anxious people are often the most creative because they are so highly aware of the world around them. Being sensitive allows you to experience the beauty around you that other people often miss because they are too busy rushing, thinking, worrying and living on autopilot.

With repeated practice of mindfulness techniques, this relaxed state can become a long-term character trait because of the changes in brain function and structure that occur during mindful practice. The brain changes in response to experience. So any repeated experience, good or bad, will create a lasting impression in the brain, which affects the way we think and behave and respond. Changing your life means changing your experience, which includes where you focus your attention.

John Teasdale, a leading mindfulness researcher, says:

> Mindfulness is a habit, it's something the more one does, the more likely one is to be in that mode with less and less effort... it's a skill that can be learned. It's accessing something we already have. Mindfulness isn't difficult. What's difficult is to remember to be mindful.

The benefits of mindfulness

Practising mindfulness has been clinically proven to reduce stress, blood pressure, depression, anxiety and addictive behaviours, and has also been proven to help people sleep better, work more effectively and improve their personal and professional relationships. Mindfulness gives you more awareness of your own feelings, thoughts and beliefs, and improves attention and concentration.

Mindful deep-breathing exercises can reduce anxiety, insomnia, depression and other ailments. It also raises the levels of hormones in the brain that make you feel good, such as oxytocin and dopamine, and lowers the level of cortisol, the hormone released by stress. When you breathe deeply, you experience better mental clarity, focus and attention and concentration.

Researchers from Texas Tech University looked at the impact that short-term meditation has on the brain and found that after 11 hours of training over a 4-week period, the mind–body participants scored significantly lower on tests for anger and hostility, confusion, depression, fatigue and total mood disturbance compared with the control group.

Further studies reveal the following benefits of practising mindfulness:

- Researchers from the University of New Mexico found that participation in a mindfulness-based stress reduction (MBSR) course decreased anxiety and binge eating.
- Office workers who practised MBSR for 20 minutes a day reported an average 11 per cent reduction in perceived stress.

- Eight weeks of MBSR resulted in an improvement in the immune profiles of people with breast or prostate cancer, which corresponded with decreased depressive symptoms.
- A prison offering Vipassana meditation training for inmates found that those who completed the course showed lower levels of drug use, greater optimism and better self-control.
- Ten-year-old girls who completed a 10-week programme of yoga and other mindfulness practices were more satisfied with their bodies and less preoccupied with weight.
- The likelihood of recurrence for patients who had experienced three or more bouts of depression was reduced by half through mindfulness-based cognitive therapy, an offshoot of MBSR.
- After 15 weeks of practising MBSR, counselling students reported improved physical and emotional well-being, and a positive effect on their counselling skills and therapeutic relationships.
- In a study at Wake Forest University School of Medicine in the USA, researchers found that after only 14 days of meditation training, subjects were able to improve their cognitive abilities.

By focusing on your breath in a relaxed way, you are teaching yourself to regulate your emotions by raising your awareness of mental processes as they are happening. Mindfulness meditation teaches you to let go of things that would easily distract you, whether it is your own thoughts or an external noise.

Practising mindfulness every day

With practice, mindfulness can become part of your everyday life. It should not be difficult or a chore or even time-consuming. It should be relaxing and enjoyable. It is about approaching your life in a state of calmness and acceptance, having an awareness of yourself as living in every moment, and of recognizing and appreciating the beauty and the joy that each moment can bring. Even when you are drinking a cup of tea, simply by focusing on the tea you can enjoy its aroma, its taste and the way it makes you feel. If your mind is full of anxious thoughts, you will not be able to enjoy the tea. Mindfulness is letting go of thinking and planning and worrying, and simply remembering to breathe. It is about creating moments of joy as you go through your day, instead of rushing from one moment to the next without noticing the beauty within them. Mindfulness expert Thich Nhat Hanh suggests five ways to live a more mindful life using mindful breathing techniques, and to bring those moments of joy to your day, every day:

1 *Mindful breathing*   This is a way of breathing that allows you to simply become aware of the breath you are breathing in and out. Recognize the in-breath and the out-breath as the object of your mindfulness and simply focus your attention on it. By focusing on your breathing in this way, the noise of your thoughts will disappear. Your mind will calm because your attention is focused on your breathing. You are no longer worrying about things to do or how to be. You are simply present, and as your body relaxes and your mind is cleared of tension, you will feel the happiness of such peace and freedom.

2 *Concentration*   Your mindfulness can focus on anything. It doesn't have to be your breathing, although mindful breathing benefits both your mind and your body. But concentrating on anything will allow you to develop insight into that object, whether it's a horse, a flower, yourself or someone else. Consequently, your insight will liberate you from fear, anger and despair and allow you to experience peace and happiness. Start by concentrating on your breathing. No matter how long or fast your breaths last, simply focus on them as you breathe in and as you breathe out. Think only of your breathing and concentrate. Your breathing will become deeper and slower and more peaceful, naturally.

3 *Awareness*   Breathing makes you more aware of your body. When you are aware of your body, you are centred in the present moment. Your body exists here and now, and not in the past or the future. It allows you to feel alive and to experience the joys of life all around you through your senses. Breathe in and breathe out and become aware of your body as you breathe.

4 *Releasing tension*   Becoming aware of your body allows you to notice the way your body feels. You may notice a tightness in your chest or a pain in your leg – the tension caused by stress. Stress affects the body and accumulates over time, so being unaware of the way you feel means the stress is allowed to continue to take a toll on your body, as well as your mind. You can release the tension in your body through relaxation, whether you are sitting, lying down or standing. Hanh suggests that the next time you are driving and come to a red light, sit back, relax and breathe deeply. Say to yourself,

'Breathing in, I'm aware of my body. Breathing out, I release the tension in my body.' You can do this anywhere, at any time, such as at work, or while you are doing the washing up. Breathe in and out, focus on your body and release any tension you become aware of.

5 *Walking meditation*   Walking mindfully is a way of being aware of your body and every step you take, and enjoying every step. It does not have to take any effort. When you walk with awareness of every step, every step brings healing. Every step brings peace. We'll explore walking mindfully more in Chapter 8.

Taking the time to practise mindfulness regularly will result in enormous benefits, both physically and mentally. You can begin a meditation practice or take a daily yoga class in a routine that suits you. But even when you are very busy, you can practise mindfulness. It can simply be part of the way you live your life, a life lived mindfully, a life lived so that you are aware of your life.

You may not have time for formal practice or a class when you have a full-time job and small children. But the real practice of mindfulness is simply to be fully in the present. When you are with your children, be with them fully. When you are putting them to bed or getting them ready for school, don't rush in an effort to get on with your life. Those moments *are* your life.

Simply by being present, by listening and being aware, of noticing others' feelings and responses as well as your own, you will gain insight into your loved ones, yourself and your relationship and an even deeper understanding, compassion and love.

You can choose to be fully present in whatever you do. Spending your life doing things you enjoy, things that are meaningful to you, will allow you to focus on the present moment and concentrate more easily on what you are doing because it resonates with a special part of you and you won't be wishing you were doing something else. If you work as a bank clerk, for example, and feel bored and frustrated, take notice. If you only allow yourself to do things you enjoy, such as painting watercolours, when you are on holiday and yet you feel relaxed, fulfilled, peaceful and happy when you do, take notice. Become aware of the things that inspire and fulfil you, and the way that certain activities make you feel. The tasks that fill you with peace and joy are the things you should be doing. You are meant to spend your life doing things that make you happy and relaxed, and noticing the joy that lives in your heart.

7

Developing awareness, facing your feelings

Facing your feelings can be frightening, intimidating and overwhelming. But your feelings will not hurt you. They are there to help you, to guide you in the right direction, away from untruths and judgements and towards acceptance and love for yourself.

Trying to cope with fear and other feelings by avoiding, denying or suppressing them is like living in a house full of clutter and telling yourself that the house is tidy, even as you are tripping over boxes and losing things you once held dear. The reality is that the clutter doesn't go away just because you are not aware of it. It continues to affect your life in an increasingly restricting way. You keep adding to it every time you deny its existence, filling every room until you can hardly find the space to breathe.

Living in a clean and tidy house means cleaning up the mess and throwing out all the stuff you no longer want or need. Shoving it all in the closet won't help. The only way to make room for the things you want in your life, and to get rid of the stuff that you don't want, is to accept what is there. And mindfulness can help you see what is right in front of you.

Of course, house cleaning is no easy task, especially if you have never done it before. Just the thought of it can be overwhelming, intimidating and scary. Many people avoid facing their feelings because of fear. Some people fear facing their emotions because they worry about the negative consequences of experiencing their own feelings, or what has been called fear of emotion. Other researchers have suggested that some people feel threatened by emotion because they associate emotional states with losing control and ultimately losing their identity.

Why should feelings be such a threat to our sense of identity? In a further study, scientists found that there is a distinct view of achievement in Western culture, which involves gaining control of one's surroundings and consequently subduing emotions. Eastern culture, conversely, places greater emphasis on seeking harmony between the individual and society. Control is highly valued in Western society, largely due to the emphasis on the individual rather than the group. Western culture also views emotion as a reflection of chaos and lack of control, which many people find frightening because they feel it prevents them from predicting their own actions, others' responses, or their own future. Emotion is often seen as an outside force that becomes a 'threatening intruder' to a person's sense of self and self-control. But researchers have discovered that avoidance and suppression as strategies for coping with emotions are linked to psychopathology and that fear of emotions can lead to prolonged negative mood states.

While denying painful feelings can feel like the right and natural thing to do sometimes, what we really need is a balance between control and acceptance. It's healthy to be able to predict certain outcomes in life and to feel in control over your own life. But it's also healthy to let go and simply accept things as they are. Dealing with your feelings does not mean that you control them by keeping them at bay. It's about accepting them. They are there for a reason, to alert you to what may be troubling you, and to allow you to take the necessary action to deal with the root problem.

How mindfulness can help

A study by Kirk Brown revealed that people who scored highly on a mindfulness scale had more control over their thinking, their behaviour and their expression. Mindfulness allows you to become more aware of the world around you, as well as the way you think and behave, and develop a non-judgemental awareness of your feelings, giving you more direction over your own life. You begin to notice that you are worrying or that you are feeling fearful or angry, and you can shift your focus to the present moment and relax. That kind of self-directed thinking consequently decreases stress, lowers anxiety and builds the self-confidence that will carry you forward.

Mindfulness meditation not only relaxes you and makes you more focused on the present, but it also increases brain activity in the prefrontal cortex, the area in the brain associated with positive emotion. People who are depressed often show less activity in this area.

Mindfulness helps you to develop a detached observance of your feelings, which can lead to insight and understanding about yourself.

Instead of *reacting* to thoughts, feelings or external stimulation like noise or other people, mindfulness teaches you to simply *observe* your thoughts and feelings and become aware of them as they emerge. In this way, you can maintain the emotional distance that allows you to avoid becoming overwhelmed or absorbed by them.

Additionally, it teaches you to recognize patterns in your thinking and behaviour, such as noticing that you become fearful every time your boyfriend tells you he is going on a business trip. Your emotional response feels familiar, but it results in repeated patterns of behaviour. You can catch yourself doing things, such as becoming angry, and choose to step in and change the course of your actions. When you become aware of your anger, for example, you can stop and ask yourself, 'Why am I so angry?', which has a tendency not only to dissolve the intensity of the emotion, but allow you to feel relaxed enough to reflect and open your mind up to possible alternative behaviours and ways of thinking.

> Penny had always been anxious about work. She knew she didn't like making presentations, but she had assumed it was because she wasn't very good at them and that she simply had to put up with the painful feelings they caused. But she has since learned to become more aware of her physical symptoms of anxiety, including sweating hands and a dry mouth, and the feelings of fear that arise at these times. She recognizes that the fear is caused by her thoughts of making a mistake in the presentation and embarrassing herself. But instead of worrying and imagining the worst-case scenario, she takes a break when she feels afraid and makes a cup of tea, allowing herself to become aware of the feelings that come up as if she were watching birds settle on a tree branch. She asks herself what she is really so afraid of, and as she sips her tea and calms down, she realizes that she is afraid of failing to do her job properly. She is afraid of failing. Her father had always told her that she could not fail in school or she would be letting him down. And that belief had become embedded in her subconscious mind, deep down where she was unaware of it, but she felt the effects of its presence nonetheless.

> Recognizing that that thought – which is only a thought – had caused her anxiety makes her feel better. It is only a thought. Fear is only a feeling. And the beliefs that caused it are part of her past. Now she can live in the present. Even if she makes a mistake, she will not be a failure. She sips her tea and focuses on the present moment, savouring the flavour of the tea, enjoying the aroma. She takes a deep breath and pays attention to each breath coming in and out. In her mind, she

watches the birds fly out of the tree, as her painful feelings fly away with them. Simply seeing that her old beliefs and her thoughts, which she no longer wants, have made her feel bad allows her to look at them from a distance, as tangible and transient objects, and let them be until they simply lose their hold on her and fade away.

Becoming mindful of the subconscious mind

Emotions are triggered by our thoughts, many of which are unconscious. When we are unconscious or unaware of our thoughts, we tend to react in an instinctive way – as if we are confronted by a potential threat. But the reaction is often inappropriate to the actual circumstances, because of the feelings that have been triggered. Once you are able to become detached from those feelings and observe them without becoming involved in them, you will be less likely to become triggered by an automatic and emotional reaction.

If you think of your mind as a bus and you are on the road of life, your subconscious is the driver. And you are the passenger. This is why we often end up in situations or with certain kinds of people or repeating things without really knowing why. We don't want them, but they keep happening. You can certainly make conscious decisions and choices about your life every day, from what to wear to where to go for dinner to whom to have a relationship with. But the choices are often based on your own subconscious beliefs, assumptions, attitudes and perspectives. Jon Kabat-Zinn explains:

> While our thinking colours all our experience, more often than not our thoughts tend to be less than completely accurate. Usually they are merely uninformed private opinions, reactions and prejudices based on limited knowledge and influenced primarily by our past conditioning.

The subconscious also creates dreams, hopes, joys and fears, which can push us towards our goals or drive us to self-defeating behaviour. So it's important to distinguish between the subconscious stories we tell ourselves, the stories we believe, and the conscious effects those beliefs have on our lives. By becoming aware of your subconscious thoughts, you can draw the focus of your attention into your conscious mind and learn to recognize the thoughts, beliefs and fears that are controlling your life. Once you are aware of them, you can choose which ones to keep, such as your belief that everyone deserves a second chance, and which ones to let go, such as your fear that you don't deserve that chance.

Mindfulness can help you to step out of negative subconscious thinking into mindful awareness, into the present moment. You can gain control of your life instead of living in fear and wondering how you got there. It's a matter of becoming aware that there are unconscious and conscious processes at work.

Because mindfulness helps you to become more aware, you can recognize with greater clarity the daily events of your life and the internal and external influences upon you. And awareness naturally moves those influences, assumptions, thoughts, beliefs, behaviour and feelings out of your subconscious and into your conscious mind, where you can *choose* how you want to respond to them.

Developing your emotional awareness

Learning to become aware of your feelings and deal with them effectively is not a personality trait that only certain people are born with, but skills that anyone can learn. These skills involve identifying, experiencing and accepting your emotions. Using these skills, you can help to clear the path for self-understanding and move from past, subconscious behaviour towards present awareness, peace and happiness. When you turn towards your feelings instead of pushing them away, you will begin to accept them not as negative experiences to be thwarted, but useful signs pointing you in the right direction. In this way, emotional awareness allows you to help yourself live a life of peace, harmony, love and compassion.

Psychotherapist Miriam Greenspan says:

Attending to, befriending and surrendering to fear, we find the courage to open to our vulnerability and we are released into the joy of knowing that we can live with and use our fear wisely. Attending to, befriending and surrendering to despair, we discover that we can look into the heart of darkness in ourselves and our world, and emerge with a more resilient faith in life.

Psychologist Jerry Duvinsky, author of *How to Lose Control and Gain Emotional Freedom: Embracing the 'Dark' Emotions Through Integrative*

Mindful Exposure, offers a mindfulness technique called 'emotional surfing', based on the idea that you cannot fight or avoid emotions any more than you can fight or avoid a wave. Instead, you must ride them out. By identifying, experiencing and accepting your feelings, you will be able to ride the waves of emotion back to shore. Here's how:

- Focus upon and hold a painful image, memory, thought or feeling.
- Label as specifically as possible the feeling(s) that arise.
- Take note and hold your attention at the bodily area from where the present feelings emanate.
- Pay careful attention to how the emotions, images and physical sensations change and move as you maintain focus. The feelings will soon pass.

Self-soothing is another important part of developing your emotional awareness. Many people shy away from experiencing their own feelings because they are painful and make us uncomfortable. But knowing how to soothe yourself means you can face those feelings and still feel okay. Soothing yourself means that you face painful memories with empathy and compassion for yourself. You are not only calming yourself but accepting yourself, which opens the door for change. You do not need to change who you are, but only the ways you think and behave that bring you distress. Change is not easy, however, so it's important to realize that it is going to take time and you need to be gentle with yourself.

Loving-kindness meditation is a type of meditation that focuses on generating open-mindedness and positive emotions such as love and compassion. Researchers have suggested that even temporary experiences of positive emotions can lead to enduring personal traits over time, which in turn can foster improved physical health as well as greater happiness in relationships and at work. The result is that positive emotions lead people to develop personal resources which improve their life satisfaction.

Repressed feelings build up over time, often leading to feelings of anxiety, fear and anger. While these feelings are generated by specific thoughts, the accumulation of painful feelings will also exacerbate those feelings and create the sensation of being overwhelmed, which can lead to depression. The key is to tackle your feelings one at a time, as they occur. Learn to become aware of them by listening to your body's response, such as an increased heart rate or sweaty palms or the realization that you are shouting. Don't judge yourself harshly for these reactions. Just listen to them. And then ask yourself, 'What am I afraid of? Why am I so angry?' If you remain quiet and let go of the talking in your head, the answers will rise to the surface of your mind. Penny, for example, found herself hearing the words 'you're going to fail' whenever she became anxious. She knew those were words her father had said to her and she decided to no longer listen or believe them. This is not about blaming yourself or anyone else for your feelings. Simply knowing why you are feeling the way you are feeling can provide enormous relief, as well as build your self-esteem because you were able to help yourself, understand yourself and accept yourself and your feelings.

It was not easy for Penny to know that her father felt that way about her or that she felt that way about herself. But she realized she now had a choice. So instead of fighting those thoughts or trying to push them away, thereby stirring up more painful feelings, she accepted them for what they were, let herself feel them, and then watched them go. She could then decide how to behave. One of the benefits of emotions is that they give us energy to act. They are there to compel us and drive us forward towards personal transformation.

But there is nothing wrong with reaching out to others for help. Emotional awareness and soothing also can come in the form of acceptance and validation of your feelings by someone else. A recent study in the journal *Psychological Science* revealed that fearful people who talked about their feelings when they were experiencing a frightening situation were better able to manage their feelings and behaviour over time. The mutual understanding and empathy that can arise from open validation and compassion can provide a sense of security as well as lasting positive emotions, well-being and self-esteem.

The more you become aware of your emotions and face them, talk about them, accept them and understand them, the more easily they will speak to you in ways that will allow you to flourish. Soon you will be aware of which emotions you are feeling and why they are there without even trying. They will simply be, and you will have developed emotional wisdom, courage, self-respect, compassion, empathy and a deeper understanding of yourself that you can lean on in difficult times and celebrate in times of joy.

8

Mindful eating, mindful walking

Why do so many of us struggle with eating and exercise? We love food, and yet it fails to bring us the happiness we crave. We rush through meals and don't pay attention to what or how we are eating. Instead of fuelling our bodies with nutrients, we are often creating negative feelings such as fear, anxiety, irritability or depression because of the foods we eat, such as sugar, fat, salt, caffeine and processed foods. We end up depressed, fatigued or host to any number of illnesses, including fibromyalgia, chronic fatigue syndrome, diabetes, heart disease and cancer.

A recent study in the journal *BMC Medicine* revealed that processed meats such as bacon, ham, sausage and salami increase the risk of cardiovascular disease, cancer and even early death. The researchers said that the salt and chemicals used to preserve the meat may damage health, and that people who eat processed meat are also more likely to smoke and to be overweight, which lead to further health problems.

We likewise need exercise, but we often see it as a chore and end up simply going through the motions without enjoying the experience. More often, we don't exercise at all and both our physical and mental health suffers.

The problem is that we are often eating and exercising mindlessly. We blame our genes, our upbringing or lack of time for our weight problems and health issues and continue to engage in unhealthy habits. Eating and exercising mindfully means that you are aware of the way your body responds to the food you eat and the way you move and that you allow yourself to slow down and enjoy these activities as they happen. A mindful approach will benefit not only your health but your mental well-being as well, giving you the peace of mind and the strength to take control of your health and deal with the fears that so often affect it.

Eating mindfully

Mindful eating means paying attention to what you are eating and the way it makes you feel, including the smell of your food, its colours and textures, the variety of flavours, and the temperatures and sensations that food stimulates within us. Do certain foods make you feel more relaxed or more energized? Do some foods make you sleepy while others increase your anxiety? Are you feeling hungry or are you thirsty, or perhaps depressed or bored? How do you know when you have had enough? Not paying attention to your eating can easily result in consuming meals without noticing what or how much you have actually eaten and not even enjoying what you did eat.

Studies by the US National Institutes of Health show that mindfulness can help you lose weight by regulating eating patterns, decreasing binges and helping you metabolize food faster. A study in the *Journal of the American Dietetic Association* found that women who ate their meals slowly ate fewer calories and drank more water than when they ate faster. They were also more likely to feel satiated when they ate slowly.

Of course, eating slowly is not a weight loss solution for everyone. If you have a condition such as leptin resistance, your body is physically less aware of feeling full and more prone to feeling the need to eat at the smell or sight of food. Likewise, research shows that poor eating habits as a child can fool your brain into thinking that unhealthy foods, such as sugar, salt and fat, are the most rewarding. Cheese, for example, produces a chemical that blocks the satiety awareness in your brain and increases cravings.

But eating mindfully will help you to become aware of the effects of certain foods on your body and the way they make you feel emotionally. It allows you to not only enjoy everyday experiences, such as the pleasure of preparing a meal and sharing it with loved ones, but to recognize the effects of food on both your body and your mind, so *you* can decide which ones to choose and take control of your life.

There is no right or wrong way to eat, but becoming aware of the way that certain foods make you feel is important to your well-being, as is the effect that rushing through a meal has on your physical and emotional health. What you eat, how you eat and how you prepare food is up to you. When you pay attention to food in the present moment, rather than forcing yourself to diet for the long-term benefits, you are able to enjoy food every day and make healthy choices at every meal. By taking a mindful approach to food, you will begin to pay attention to your thoughts, feelings and bodily sensations. You will notice the behaviours you have adopted about food that have not served you well and the ones that do.

Another key element of mindfulness that also applies to mindful eating is not to judge yourself. Many of us have learned unhealthy ways of eating or dealing with our emotions, and they become habits so ingrained we are not even aware of them. Mindfulness allows you to bring that awareness to the table. And it allows you to accept your past behaviours without self-criticism or blame, and to simply acknowledge that they exist knowing that you now have the opportunity to change your behaviours if you want to.

Because mindful eating includes eating more slowly, you can enjoy your food more. But enjoyment does not mean that you will eat more. In fact, the slower you eat, the less you eat. But you will still feel full when you have eaten the right amount for your body. Eating slowly gives your body the time it needs, which is about 20 minutes, to digest the food and signal the brain when it has had enough. Eat faster than this and you will consume more than you need. You will also enjoy it less.

Many of us have a fear that causes us to eat as quickly as possible, such as the fear that someone will take the food away, or that we won't get as much as our siblings, or the fear that we'll miss some special event if we don't eat quickly. But as an adult, you can remind yourself that you have enough time. Eat slowly and enjoy it. No one will steal your food. You will have enough. And you won't miss anything. You will simply experience the pleasure of it.

Here are some further suggestions for eating mindfully:

- Think about whether or not you are actually hungry before you start to eat.
- Create a calming place for enjoying meals. Set the table with candles, flowers or your favourite tablecloth and turn on relaxing music to create a calming atmosphere and a sense of pleasure and appreciation for the food you are eating.
- Set aside at least 20 minutes for meal times. Try using a timer.
- Avoid watching TV, reading or surfing the Internet while you are eating, as these distractions will keep you from enjoying your food and prevent your awareness of how much you are eating.

- Eat small but frequent meals to avoid feeling too hungry or too full. Protein and fibre-rich foods will help to keep you feeling satisfied. And knowing that you can eat again in 2 or 3 hours means you don't have to overfill yourself at one meal.
- Put your utensils down between bites and chew your food thoroughly.
- Listen to your body and notice how full you are feeling. Eating slowly will give you time to notice your body. Once you feel full, stop eating. Eating according to the way you feel will help you to become aware of your own appetite.

Janet was an 'emotional eater'. She used food not to provide her body with nutrients but to calm herself down when she felt afraid. She ate so quickly that she could polish off a litre of ice cream in front of the TV without even realizing it. What's worse, she hadn't even tasted it after the first bite. Unhappy with her health and her weight, as well as her persistent fears and insecurities, Janet began to ask herself why she was eating junk food. She knew she ate when she felt scared or worried. She came to realize that she was using food to fill a void inside her that opened up whenever she was worried. And she became worried when she thought that someone she loved was in danger. So she realized that she ate mindlessly when her children came home late from school, or when they didn't call. And when her husband hurt his back in an accident she ate constantly, as if she could stuff her feelings down and fill up the worry and fear with food. The trouble was that while her stomach was full, her heart was still aching with need. Food, she realized, wasn't going to fill that need, no matter what or how much she ate.

Psychologist Susan Albers, author of *Eating Mindfully: How to End Mindless Eating and Enjoy a Balanced Relationship with Food*, notes that for many of us, eating is a way of coping with our emotions. But like Janet discovered, eating this way – mindlessly – is only a temporary fix, and eating to deal with our feelings only helps us to avoid facing and processing those feelings and consequently we end up feeling worse.

Mindfulness practices such as meditation, yoga and journalling can help you to become more aware of your feelings, and to recognize and identify them. The more you try to avoid your feelings, the bigger they will become and that's what often makes us feel hopeless, fearful and victimized. Face your feelings and express them either by writing about them or talking to someone trustworthy. Once you get your feelings out, you will feel not only relieved but empowered, and then you can begin to change the thought patterns that led to those feelings and develop a more positive perspective on your life, your eating habits and yourself. Remember, be gentle with yourself. Don't feel bad or guilty about your feelings. They are there to guide you.

Exercise

Any kind of exercise will help to reduce your fear and anxiety and build your self-esteem while flooding your body with oxygen, improving circulation and heart health, and burning calories. Exercise is also one of the best stress relievers because it increases your feelings of calm and elevates mood. Research shows that exercise can help to alleviate depression. In fact, a study in *Psychosomatic Medicine* revealed that the benefits of exercise are comparable to antidepressants.

When it comes to dealing with fear, exercise is also an effective coping method. Fear triggers our nervous system, creating reactions such as sweating, a pounding heart and shaking hands, and we can respond to those symptoms with more fear. But since exercise produces a lot of the same reactions, including pounding heart and sweating, researchers found that people who exercised regularly reduced their sense of fear and anxiety. In the study, exercise acted like exposure therapy, so that participants came to associate the symptoms of a racing heart and sweating with something positive rather than with fear.

Regular exercise can even protect from the effects of stress in the future, as it helps you to develop resistance to the stress hormone cortisol. In addition, exercise produces endorphins, the chemicals in the brain that create the 'runner's high', which act like natural painkillers as well as improve sleep quality.

Walking mindfully

Walking is an excellent form of exercise, and mindful walking is a form of mindfulness that allows your body to move while you meditate, so that you can focus on your movements and live in the present moment as a way of letting go of your thoughts and developing your awareness. By becoming aware of your feet touching the ground, you develop a mind–body connection as well as a sense of connection to the earth that is very calming and helps to reduce stress.

The idea of mindful walking is not to reach a destination but to focus on the walk, so practitioners often choose a circular walk or simply walk to one point and back again. Labyrinths have been used in many cultures for thousands of years to help quiet and focus the mind as part of the spiritual journey. The natural spiral pattern reminds you of nature as you walk towards the centre, and the highly symbolic nature of labyrinths inspires a sense of wholeness, the journey to one's inner self and back out to the world again, and the path we walk in life.

Research by scientists at Harvard's Mind/Body Institute shows that walking a labyrinth can provide long-term health benefits, in part because it promotes relaxed brain-wave activity. This relaxed state enhances creativity and problem-solving abilities and encourages self-understanding, as well as promoting the feeling of centredness. The balance created between mind and body by walking mindfully, and the state of calm and groundedness generated, frees you from the frenetic thinking that so often populates our minds. It creates a space for insights and inner knowledge from both the conscious and unconscious minds to rise effortlessly to the surface, helping you to respond to life's demands.

Mindfulness expert Thich Nhat Hahn suggests ways to benefit from mindful walking in his book *Peace Is Every Step: The Path of Mindfulness in Everyday Life*. Here's how:

- Start your walk with the intention to walk mindfully, whether it's to develop your awareness, increase feelings of calm or reduce stress. If you are walking a labyrinth, think of where you are in your life and be open to whatever comes to you as you walk. The intention is not to seek answers, however, but to calm your mind and your body.
- Walking outdoors in a quiet, natural setting will provide the added calming influence of nature.
- As you begin, become aware of your feet touching the ground and the muscles moving in your legs. Feel the sensation of the ground beneath your feet.
- As you walk, notice your environment. What are the sights, sounds and smells you notice?
- Expand your awareness so that you notice your thoughts and the way you feel, physically and emotionally. Do you like the way a

breeze tousles your hair? Do the trees stir up childhood memories and feelings? Do you feel energized or relaxed? Remember to breathe.

• Remember not to judge your thoughts or feelings or experiences, but simply to notice them and turn your focus back to the present moment and your walking.

By incorporating mindful walking and mindful eating into your life, you are bringing a sense of peace and calm into your daily activities that may not have previously existed. These mindfulness practices take some repetition to reap the most benefits, but the relaxation, creativity, confidence and calm they add to your life will flow into all your activities, even when you are not practising. The fear that has consumed you will begin to release its hold on you, so that you are no longer feeling afraid or victimized or depressed by the lack of control over your own life. And the insights you gain from these simple meditations will provide you with the knowledge and insights deep inside you that can help you to see where you have stumbled and how to get back on your feet. Your body will be nourished, not overfed, your heart and mind will be clear and creative, and the awareness that you have brought into your life will make your spirit soar.

9

Meditation and yoga

Mindfulness is a state of mind, a way of being, and it takes practice to achieve this state of mind. It's not a personality trait or an ability that some of us have and some don't. Overcoming fear through mindfulness is a skill that anyone can learn and, over time, the benefits of practising such skills produce results in the same way that regular exercise tones your body. Mindfulness practices enable you to enter that state of awareness and non-judgement and cultivate a greater awareness in your everyday life. Meditation and yoga are two important mindfulness practices that can help you to open the door to a mindful life.

Meditation and yoga are mind–body practices that focus on attention to what you are doing in the present moment without judgement, fostering mental well-being, including calmness, clarity and concentration, which in turn contribute to the ability to control one's own emotions. Mind–body practices are effective because the body and mind affect each other. When you are thinking negative thoughts, you begin to feel angry or upset and then your body begins to respond accordingly, pumping blood through your veins, creating a tightness in your jaw or a knot in your stomach. Likewise, when your back aches and your head is throbbing, your mind turns to thoughts and feelings of dismay, discouragement and depression. Mindfulness practices allow the body and mind to work together to gain mental clarity, relaxation and improved physical and mental health.

Fear can be debilitating because it is driven by negative thoughts, which in turn create unpleasant feelings, as well as anxiety, depression and physical symptoms. By focusing your attention on the present moment, you can allow yourself to become aware of those negative thoughts and inner fears, and let them go.

Benefits

Mindfulness meditation has been shown to benefit both the mind and the body in many ways, including boosting the immune system, reducing blood pressure and improving cognitive function. Researchers have found that these positive effects are due to the four key elements of mindfulness, which work together to help us cope with stress in gentle and non-judgemental ways: attention regulation, body awareness, emotion regulation and sense of self.

Because mindfulness practices encourage awareness of your thoughts, feelings and your body, you will develop an increasing recognition of when your body or your mind are out of sync. When previously you may not have even been aware that you were walking bent over because your back was sore, mindfulness allows you to notice your back and your posture, and the thoughts and feelings that are affecting it, while empowering you to control those thoughts and feelings and your sense of well-being in a gentle, compassionate and harmonious way.

Mindfulness practice has also been shown to reduce anxiety and depression. One study showed that mindfulness meditation reduced distractive and ruminative thoughts and behaviours, which helped to reduce distress. Another study also found that mindfulness meditation helps to develop self-observation skills, which disengage the automatic pathways in the brain created by prior learning and allow new information to be integrated. In this way, we are able to adapt more easily and positively to stressful situations.

Many studies have found that the focused breathing used in meditation practices provides improved emotional responses and lowers stress by enabling the selective experience of emotion. Further studies have shown that mindfulness practices improve focus and attention and consequently decrease emotional reactivity, increase immune function and foster a greater sense of relaxation and compassion for oneself and others. The mindfulness skills of adapting to stress and being aware of and communicating your emotions can also have positive effects on your relationships.

The benefits of mindfulness practice are endless, but essentially they enable you to strengthen your ability to *choose* where you put your attention. This kind of self-awareness is achieved through various means during mindfulness practice, including reducing negative thoughts, regulating your behaviour and increasing positive feelings about yourself and others.

Meditation

There are many different types of meditation, with different intentions, but mindful meditation focuses on developing your awareness of the present moment without judgement. You will not be 'zoned out' or in some trance-like state, but simply calm and aware.

Sitting in a comfortable position, close your eyes and simply notice the sensations in your body, your feelings and the thoughts in your mind without judging them as good or bad or having to do something about them. Just be aware of them. As these thoughts and feelings and sensations come and go, you will gradually be able to quiet your mind and feel a greater sense of calm as you separate yourself from these transitory experiences.

While you are becoming aware of what is happening in the moment, focus your attention on your breathing. When you notice a thought or a feeling or a physical sensation, you can acknowledge it and then bring your attention back to your breathing, a technique known as 'touch and go'.

What you are trying to achieve is a state of calm, without attaching any judgement, blame, criticism, shame, resentment or any other attitude to your thoughts or feelings. Recognize that they simply exist like clouds and watch them pass by. Breathing mindfully will help you to refocus your attention from these clouds back onto the present moment. With practice, your mind will achieve a natural state of calm without effort, just as with physical exercise you can train your body to run without struggling.

The goal of meditation is not to become a champion meditator but to experience the increasing sense of calm and relaxation that you bring to your life, the compassion and empathy that appears in your relationships with others and the loving acceptance you have with yourself.

Before you begin your meditation practice, there are a few conditions that will help you to train your mind more effectively:

- Find a place to meditate that will allow you to relax and feel calm, even if it is just a corner of a room. The space should be quiet and allow you to be uninterrupted, and should not trigger any negative thoughts or feelings.

- Your meditation practice should be frequent but short. Ten or 15 minutes in the morning and again in the evening can give your mind time to develop gently.

- When you first sit down, you cannot expect your mind to simply take you away. You must concentrate. Take a deep breath and tell yourself that you are here to train your mind. Begin with the intention to attain mindfulness.

- Meditation is a mind–body practice which means that one affects the other. Be sure that your posture is relaxed but upright and not slouched or bent over, and keep your feet flat on the ground if you are sitting in a chair. Place your hands in any position that is comfortable for you. Give yourself a moment to feel your body and settle into a stable, erect posture. If you begin to fall asleep, readjust your posture.

- You can keep your eyes open or closed. If open, focus downward slightly while keeping your head up. You are not meant to be staring at anything, but simply minimizing sensory stimulation.

- Focus on your breathing as you allow thoughts and feelings to flow in and out of your mind. The benefit of focusing on your breathing, as opposed to focusing on an object in front of you, is that breathing naturally relaxes you.

- When you become aware of a thought or feeling, tell yourself that you are aware of it and you are letting it go because now is not the time to think about it. Now is the time to breathe. You will see how fast your thoughts come and go, and that is part of what creates feelings of fear and anxiety. Meditation helps you to slow your mind down, giving you an increased feeling of calm.

Since mindful meditation is meant to be a journey, not a destination, we can often experience obstacles along the way, such as distractions, boredom, fear or frustration. It can also be hard to change old habits and let go of negative beliefs. But as with any obstacles in life, you can either surrender to them or you can see them as signs along your path, increasing your awareness of your own needs and issues and refocusing your attention and motivation.

Techniques

There are many different ways of practising mindfulness meditation, but here are a few ways to focus your attention and bring a sense of calm and acceptance into your thinking and enhance your well-being:

Focused attention meditation   Focus on your breath as it enters your body and then leaves. After a minute or two, shift your attention to the sounds you hear around you, or any other sensation in your body, including the sound of your own breathing. While this technique is relaxing, the goal of this meditation is simply to be present.

Open presence meditation   Begin with focused attention meditation and then observe any thoughts or feelings that you become aware of. Allow them to simply rise to the surface and take note of their presence, neither pushing them away nor obsessing about them. Then let them pass away, just as the breath comes into the body and leaves again. In this way you experience anything that comes into your awareness without judging it or controlling it.

Loving-kindness meditation   Also known as *maitri*, this meditation is meant to generate a sense of love and compassion for oneself and others. *Maitri* means loving-kindness or unconditional friendliness and it can often develop as a natural result of mindfulness practice, but you can use this technique to overcome patterns of aggression or negative thinking. Just as you have learned negative beliefs and fears, you can also learn compassion, generosity and patience. Begin by thinking of someone you know and love and think warm wishes of love and happiness towards them. Then extend those feelings and thoughts towards other people and then even to people you do not like, and eventually to everyone. This meditation usually involves the four mantras: 'May you be safe; May you be happy; May you be healthy; May you be at ease'. You can also direct this loving mantra to yourself and say, 'May I be safe; May I be happy' and so on. By opening our hearts and offering love to others, we are offering love to ourselves. To love others, we must first nurture ourselves with gentle, loving compassion. You may not like all the thoughts and feelings that you become aware of, but you do not have to blame or criticize yourself. You can still love yourself.

Yoga

So much of what we experience emotionally, such as fear, anger, anxiety, despair and love, is experienced and stored physically, in the body. Yoga is a mind–body mindfulness practice that allows you to experience your emotions, your world, through your body, and to heal yourself through your body. As well as developing physical skills such as flexibility and strength, yoga bridges the mind and body to cultivate mindfulness skills such as patience and awareness in an environment that can also bridge the self to others.

Meditation and yoga blend harmoniously together because they both combine the mind and the body, increasing your awareness of both as they work together. By bringing mindful meditation into yoga practice, you are better able to deal with your feelings, your thoughts and your personal struggles. Your beliefs influence your thoughts, which influence your feelings, which affect your body. Whatever is in your mind you bring to your body, and vice versa. Any extreme determination to avoid either emotions or physicality will impede either process, like rocks in the road.

In yoga practice, the idea is to relax. This includes relaxing whatever thoughts, feelings, attitudes, beliefs or motives you are bringing to the session. All of it settles within your body, in your muscles and your skin, in your breathing and your heart. The Sanskrit word for posture is *asana* or 'to sit with what comes up'. That is what yoga is. It allows you to sit with what comes up with you, physically and emotionally.

Practising a physical mindfulness technique allows you to become aware of your physical presence and the effect that your feelings have on you. You might notice that you hold your breath when you are afraid or anxious. Perhaps your heart beats faster. And perhaps over time, with practice, you begin to notice that by taking deep breaths and remaining calm in the face of your own fears you can breathe deeply and slow your heart rate down, and feel not the anxious pulse of worry but the calm and unhurried breath of serenity. In this way you create not only a relaxed mind but a relaxed and contented body.

In the same way that you focus on your breathing in meditation, you focus on your breathing in yoga practice, allowing it to shift and change as you move and creating an awareness of how your breathing, and your thoughts and feelings, shift and change in your everyday life as well, coming and going with your thoughts and the obstacles you face every day. Yoga also develops your skill in patience, compassion and love, for your own strengths and weaknesses, for yourself and others.

Likewise, while there are obstacles to face in meditation, like the frustration or helplessness or lack of self-confidence that often arises when you are beginning a mindfulness practice, yoga can present obstacles as we face frustrations with ourselves or the practice or perhaps fear that we are not performing correctly, that our bodies are not responding appropriately or in the right way. Yoga, however, is about balance, between mind and body, and between active and receptive forces. Most people don't have the strength, coordination or concentration to do complex yoga moves at first, but that doesn't matter. What is important is to do the postures that come naturally and move gently forward.

Just as the breath and blood flow freely throughout the body when we move, our feelings can circulate more freely when our body is loose and the mind is open. We can accept our feelings and our thoughts and let them move on without judgement or impediment. If you are feeling afraid, or anxious or angry or sad, these feelings will show themselves in your body, through slumped shoulders, a pounding heart, an aching back or sore feet. Breathing deeply through movement will allow not only oxygen to move in and out of your body, but your feelings as well, while fuelling your muscles and your mind with the air they need to function properly.

Loving-kindness practice also applies to yoga, in what is called heart-opening poses. In these poses, you rotate your shoulders, open your ribs and do backbends that relax your chest muscles and open your heart. Again, a gentle and loving approach is key.

Poses

The following are a set of basic yoga exercises you can do that allow you to breathe, focus your mind and relax your body:

Breathe Sitting comfortably, with your posture upright, notice your breathing and the sensations in your body as you inhale and exhale.

Cat stretch Move onto your hands and knees, with your wrists directly under your shoulders and your knees under your hips. Curve your back upwards towards the ceiling and exhale, tucking your chin into your chest. As you inhale, curve your back down again, keeping the elbows straight. Repeat slowly three to five times.

Mountain pose Stand upright and draw the tailbone towards the heels, while pulling the chin down. Place the palms over your heart and breathe.

Sun salutation As you inhale, stretch your arms over your head, keeping your palms together. Exhale and move the arms to the side, then place your hands next to your feet, drawing your navel towards the base of your spine.

Downward-facing dog Inhale, then bend forward at the waist and plant your palms flat on the floor, fingers pointing forward and spread apart. If necessary, bend your knees. Step each foot back until you are in the top part of a push-up. Your hands should be beneath your shoulders with palms flat on the floor. Lift your hips towards the ceiling until your body makes an inverted 'V'. Press your chest towards your knees, keep your eyes on your toes and press your heels towards the floor. Breathe deeply.

Reclining knee to shoulder position Lie down on your back with your legs extended. Bend the right knee to the chest, clasping the shin with both hands. Tuck the chin towards the chest. Breathe and rotate the right ankle in both directions. Place the right foot on the left thigh and guide the knee towards the floor gently. Extend the right arm out and turn your head to the right. Rotate back onto your back and repeat with the left leg.

It's a good idea to end a yoga session by lying on your back with your palms turned upward. Close your eyes, relax and inhale, and concentrate on your breathing. Remember that underneath the stress and the fear and the world of emotions, lies the peace that exists always within you.

10

Journalling

The benefits of keeping a diary, or journalling, are increasingly well researched, as well as proving to be an effective way of developing your mindfulness. By giving you an outlet for your thoughts and feelings, journalling provides an arena for your voice to be heard, while silencing the critics and naysayers, including your own inner critic.

Journalling can be a form of mindful meditation because it creates an opportunity for quiet in your life and a chance to get in touch with yourself in a way that a hurried modern life often prevents. Rather than simply recording events, which has been proven to provide little benefit, mindful journalling encourages you to reflect on your thoughts and feelings, responses and perceptions about those events. By getting it all out on paper, you can clear your mind of negative self-talk and self-criticism and allow your subconscious mind to rise to the surface of your awareness, bringing forth a deep well of understanding, insight and creativity.

Jane had struggled with finding the right job and found her work as an administrative assistant depressing. She had discovered that her career didn't suit her because she was a sensitive, artistic person who needed to pursue creative activities. While she began to spend more time on the activities she enjoyed, such as gardening and drawing, she still felt frustrated and stuck in her job and it continued to make her feel depressed. Jane was a quiet and introverted person who hadn't always felt comfortable talking about her feelings, so she began writing about her job in her journal and about the way her job made her feel. She also wrote about the way gardening and drawing made her feel and what she wanted to accomplish. Over several weeks she began to become more aware of how she really felt about her work, as well as the ways that she was responding to those feelings.

Many people are hesitant to start journalling because they don't think they know how, or they don't believe they are writers, they cannot spell, or they don't have time to write. Perhaps most common are the fears that someone will read their writing or that they don't know what to write about. It's important that you don't let anyone read your journal because by keeping it private you give yourself the opportunity to express yourself freely, including the revelation of your deepest fears, anxieties, hopes and joys. You can protect your privacy by saving your journal entries on a flash drive or emailing them to your own email address. Alternatively, you can simply tear up your journal entries every day. You don't have to keep them if you don't want to. It's up to you. Knowing that no one will ever read what you are writing means that you can write with complete openness and honesty, and that is essential to bringing clarity, understanding and well-being to yourself.

> Jane's journal writing became increasingly open as she gave herself time each day to express her feelings. She also looked back over her entries and read what she had written. This process helped her to become aware that she felt more than just dissatisfied with her job. She felt depressed because she felt like a victim. She felt that she was under the control of her employer and that made her feel powerless. Recognizing the patterns in her behaviour that she had written about over time, however, made her realize that she could change the way she responded to her situation and she could change the way she felt. By writing about her experiences and her thoughts and feelings about them, Jane began to feel less victimized.

Benefits

Research by Dr James Pennebaker of the University of Texas at Austin has shown the tremendous benefits of personal writing on our physical and mental well-being. Writing about emotional topics in particular has been found to boost both your mood and your immune system. In his studies, Pennebaker found that holding in emotions created negative psychological and physical effects. By linking details to emotions through writing, however, he found that people received greater health benefits. Students who wrote about their feelings showed better grades, and workers who had been laid off found new jobs more quickly than those who did not write. Dr Pennebaker's research suggests that this kind of writing provides a release of tension, stress, frustration, hurt or anger that helps the body to withstand stress and fight off disease. A study by Joshua Smyth also found significant reduction in arthritis and asthma symptoms in patients who kept a journal.

Further studies have revealed that people who don't normally talk about their feelings, including men and people high in hostility, benefit the most from journal writing. Writing makes events and our thoughts and feelings about those events more manageable, possibly because it gives the writer a sense of control as well as a release of emotion. It can provide an accessible, safe and unrestricted outlet for expressing your feelings, which can bring forth understanding, clarity and closure. Additionally, writing in a journal can make you feel that someone is listening and that you have a confidant and a trusted friend to hear you.

How to begin journalling

How do you write in a journal in a mindful way? First, remember that it's not about creating a work of art but is instead a method of accessing your true self. Find a quiet place and a quiet time when you won't be disturbed. You will only need about 15 minutes, but try to write every day for at least 4 days in a row. The longer you write, the more you will benefit. You can write in a notebook or on a computer, in the morning or in the evening, in bed or on the bus. Write wherever and whenever feels best to you.

The important thing is not to worry about spelling or the number of words you put down. According to Pennebaker, the essence of journalling is in the way it forces you to stop rushing about and to reflect on your life. In a journal, you have permission to think about what has happened and where you want to go without criticism or complaint from anyone. For many people, just knowing that they have that time to themselves, to think about themselves and reflect, can be very therapeutic as well as a calming moment to look forward to each day.

Consider the following steps to help you begin and sustain your journal writing:

Relax Once you have found a quiet time and place, try lighting a candle or playing relaxing music. Begin with a few moments of simple meditation, like deep breathing. This will help to clear the noise in your mind and help you to quiet your mind enough to let thoughts and feelings appear naturally.

Date it If you date each journal entry you will be able to go back and read your writing with the additional benefit of seeing your own evolving thought patterns and feelings over time. You will also see where you have stopped writing and what events inspired you to start again.

Just write   When you are ready to write, don't think about what you should say or stop yourself from writing something wrong. Just write. Don't go back and change or correct your work. Let your thoughts and feelings flow naturally.

Start with feeling   Start with how you are feeling about something or relate the events like a story and capture your feelings about it afterwards.

Tell the truth   Don't worry what anyone will think. They don't need to know. But you need to be honest with yourself. This is the place to do it.

What to write about

The wonderful thing about journal writing is that you can write about anything you want. This is a space for your thoughts and feelings, your questions and reflections, your life. There are no 'shoulds' here. You can write about anything that is on your mind, such as something you are worrying about or something you are wishing for. Write about what is troubling you or what you are afraid of.

If you have not journalled before or you are not used to opening up and expressing your feelings, it can be difficult to know what to write about. In her book, *Journalution: Journaling to Awaken Your Inner Voice, Heal Your Life and Manifest Your Dreams*, author Sandy Grason suggests a few ways to get yourself writing:

Finish the sentence, 'I don't want to write about . . .'   This technique can break down your defences and get you thinking about what is really bothering you. We often try to avoid facing the real issues and fill our journal with how wonderful everything is. But if you remember that no one is going to read what you have written, you can allow yourself to tell the truth.

Answer the question, 'Who am I now?'   Think about who you were as a child compared with the person you are now. What has changed? How have you grown? And what parts of you have remained the same?

Write about things you love Sometimes we focus on the negative without stopping to consider and appreciate the positive. Write about whatever makes you feel good, whether it's a sunset, your family or the holiday you took last year.

Make a list of your good qualities You may be unaware of all the great things about yourself. When you are facing fear, it's easy to feel bad about yourself. Remind yourself on paper that you are a good person and there are plenty of things to love about you.

Have a conversation with yourself in old age What would you ask the older you? And what would the older you tell the younger you?

In his research, Pennebaker gave writing participants instructions on what and how to write. He asked people to write about their deepest thoughts and feelings about an extremely important emotional issue that had affected them. He suggested to people to really let go and explore their emotions, and possibly relate their subject to their relationships with others as well as to who they might have been, who they would like to be or who they are now. He recommended writing for a specified time and to simply keep writing until the time was up. Pennebaker found this exercise to be tremendously powerful for everyone involved. All the participants ended up expressing a huge range and depth of experiences and while many people felt sad after writing, most reported that the writing experience was valuable and meaningful to them.

> Writing put Jane in control, not only of her feelings but her life. She cringed when she reread passages she had written about how sad and helpless she was, but while it was difficult to see that side of herself, she realized that she didn't have to feel like a victim. She could see her pursuit of meaningful work as a challenge, not a defeat. She began to write about the losses she had experienced as a result of embracing the victim mentality and to separate her resentments about work from her resentments about herself and her past. She came to see that a lot of her feelings about work came from her feelings about her past and that her fear of facing those past issues and moving on was increasing her feelings of depression and self-doubt.
>
> Feeling more empowered by her journal writing, Jane was able to deal with the fears she had felt growing up and the feeling of victimization she had always felt, to the point that she stopped identifying herself as a victim and instead saw her job as only a part of her life

instead of all of it. She accepted that she had to continue working until she discovered what she wanted to do, but while she was there she would see it as a challenge and use some of the money she earned to develop her skills as an artist. Her sense of empowerment also meant that she had the strength to ask friends for help and to take the time she needed for solitude and creativity. In her journal, she wrote that she had decided to replace feeling like a victim with feeling determined.

Writing enabled her to view her situation and herself objectively, so that she could look at her life mindfully, thoughtfully and with compassion for herself. In her journalling, she was able to link her feelings with her thoughts, and to change her focus from the past to the present. In this way, she was able to take control of her life and focus on the way she wanted to feel now.

Just like any other form of mindfulness practice, journalling is not about doing it the 'right' way or evaluating your own behaviour, your writing ability or your moods. It is simply a way of becoming open and present and putting all the noise in your mind in one place while finding out who you are. You may not like what you discover about yourself on paper or how you think or feel about something or someone, but do not be hard on yourself. Mindfulness is non-judgemental. It is accepting and compassionate. And when you begin to see yourself in your journal and discover your true feelings and your true self, both good and bad, remember that you can still love yourself.

11

Mindful relationships: how to transform fear-driven feelings into love

Perhaps nowhere does fear rise to the surface of our lives more than in relationships. We fear intimacy, abandonment and commitment. We fear being alone and we fear being with the wrong person. We are afraid of getting hurt and expressing our true feelings. Sensitive people are also often easily hurt, unable to say no, take on the victim role and find it difficult to separate their own feelings from the emotions of others. And yet we are hard-wired to create meaningful connections with others. We need relationships because they teach us how to grow and become the selves we were meant to be – whole, happy and loved.

Whether the relationship is with a partner, a colleague, your parents or your children, fear is often at the root of relationship problems. Fear creates a version of you that buries your self-esteem, confuses your judgement and often attracts difficult people. But by approaching relationships mindfully, instead of fearfully, you can recover from a painful past, avoid hurtful people and find and nurture positive, loving experiences with others.

Fear-driven relationships

All relationships come with their own challenges, and learning to care for, understand and love someone and trust that the person will do the same for us is not always easy. Sensitive people have the added challenge of needing to be alone while simultaneously feeling like they are missing out. They face the challenge of wanting to be part of a community while feeling overwhelmed by group activities. They possess a drive to help others but can easily find themselves helping too much.

Whether you are an HSP or not, it's important to find the balance between self and others, between compassion and self-preservation and this comes with awareness of your own needs and feelings and the enforcement of boundaries to protect them.

Sometimes we want a relationship so badly we place our trust in the hands of people who do not deserve it and we end up getting hurt, feeling unloved and feeling bad about ourselves, as if we do not deserve a loving relationship and the cycle of attracting negative people into our lives continues.

The main reason that this pattern continues is that we are usually unaware that it is happening or that we feel badly about ourselves. It is your beliefs about yourself, such as whether you think you are a good person, whether you believe you deserve unconditional love and whether you believe it's okay to say no, that determine the kinds of relationships you will have. They can be positive or negative, but a negative belief will inevitably cause difficulties. These negative beliefs, or schemas, are powerful and not easy to change, so that even if a trusted friend tells you that your negative beliefs are not true, most people still won't change their thinking. One of the reasons they are so powerful is that we continually reinforce them by our own behaviour.

As a child, Kelly had often had to give up her own needs to look after her alcoholic father, and grew up believing that she should sacrifice her own needs for the sake of others. She wasn't even aware that she felt this way, but she behaved accordingly. As an adult, she began subconsciously to choose romantic partners who fitted her schema and she dated men who were demanding, controlling alcoholics for whom she had to sacrifice her own needs. She didn't notice that this was a problem at first because her relationships, though unhealthy, fitted the pattern of her negative belief in her mind and we are always attracted to what's familiar to us. Despite this 'fit', she became aware only that her relationships were unfulfilling and unhappy.

Many people then respond to their unhappiness by becoming angry and blaming other people, which leads to further relationship difficulties and makes any kind of growth for themselves impossible.

Brian often responded to the frustration of his own unmet needs this way. He had a demanding job, a sick mother, two kids and he and his wife had recently moved house. The pressure was getting to him and he was feeling stressed. He had always become angry when he was stressed, but as the pressure built he began arguing with his wife more often, blaming her for their money problems and for placing too many demands on him. Brian had always felt that he never really deserved his wife or the nice house they'd bought. He was dyslexic and had always been told as a boy that there was something wrong with him and he continued to believe it. So he worked harder and tried to prove to everyone that he was just as good as they were. But he didn't really believe it himself, so no matter how hard he worked or how well he provided for his family he felt inadequate, and this made him angry. What he really felt was fear. He was afraid that he was never going to be good enough for his wife or his kids or his mother, despite their loving reassurances to the contrary.

Schemas also affect relationships through pain avoidance behaviours. People subconsciously adopt certain schemas, or beliefs, and try to behave according to the rules because to defy them will mean pain and suffering. For example, Kelly believed that she should sacrifice herself for others, and the rule of that schema is that doing something for yourself will result in feeling selfish and heartless, so she avoided it. As a result, she avoided the pain of feeling selfish but she never had her needs met. She often stayed in a dysfunctional relationship because she believed she should be sacrificing herself for the other person, and leaving that relationship made her feel she was being selfish.

The key to changing your relationships is to become *aware* of what you are telling yourself and to learn to believe that you really do deserve to be loved. Ironically, the first and most important step towards finding the love you want is to love yourself. Most of the time, we approach relationships out of a sense of need. We want someone to love us, to nurture us, to give us everything that we never had growing up. Most of us carry emotional and psychological wounds from the past. And most of us feel wounded because we did not feel loved enough. When this need for love has been unfulfilled for a long time it can become desperate, anxious and fearful, and we end up entering relationships that are based on fear instead of love. Real love requires vulnerability, honesty and openness. Our own fear of getting hurt, and attempts at protecting ourselves from the hurt, manipulation, rejection or abandonment we may have felt as a child, prevent us from being open and vulnerable enough to love or be loved. Such defensive strategies undermine any possibility of real connection.

To find love, you need to be willing to face your fears. You need to learn to let go of the hurts of the past and let yourself become vulnerable and open to the possibility of love. Fear often feels safer, but it will also keep you a prisoner. To break out and live your life on your terms, it's necessary to accept the past as the past and love yourself now, the way you always wanted to be loved. Avoiding relationships, fearing intimacy or running away when a relationship becomes difficult will not bring love closer to you. It is only a way of avoiding your own fears and, ultimately, your own true self. Remember, fear won't hurt you. Face it, recognize it and it will lose its hold over you.

Unfortunately, many people in your life may try to make it harder for you to change. Your friends and family may begin to feel alienated or threatened by the new you. They may even be jealous of your new-found confidence and blossoming self-esteem and try to hold you back or sabotage your efforts. This is a risk you have to take. Becoming more confident and happy with who you are and the kind of relationships you want means that sometimes you will have to let go of relationships that are no longer working or supportive. You must root out all the messy, unpleasant beliefs and people from your past and all the hurt feelings that come with them so that you are aware of why you are afraid. And with awareness comes the freedom to make your own choices, including the choice to love and be loved.

Letting go of negative schemas is also difficult because we tend to build up evidence to support those beliefs over time. If you believe that you never do anything right, for example, you will remember experiences that support that belief. There is also plenty of evidence to contradict that belief as well, so finding the facts that support a new belief, that you do things right and well most of the time, can help weaken the strength of the old negative belief.

Likewise, while many people are aware that they are in an unhappy relationship they often feel that that is normal. Sometimes this is because they believe that they don't deserve any better, but many of us believe that love is painful, that relationships are hard work and involve sacrifice, and that to be in love is to suffer. But none of this is true. Pain and fear are not a normal part of relationships. Love is accepting and supporting and nurturing. Love helps you to grow, gently and tenderly. If love doesn't feel that way to you, it isn't love. It's probably fear.

The desire for love and romance and a committed relationship can be so strong, oftentimes because of our unfulfilled and urgent need for love, that we project our vision of love and romance onto another person without seeing them for who they really are. Again, this is a way of approaching relationships with fear because you are creating an expectation that the other person will fulfil your needs for you. By being aware not only of your own beliefs but the beliefs and needs of the other person, you can gain control of your own behaviour and choose the people and the relationships you really want.

Protecting yourself

So how do you find the relationships with family, friends, colleagues and partners that you want and avoid the ones that you don't? And how do you keep from feeling afraid and overwhelmed when you are involved with other people? The key is not to demand respect from others but to respect yourself, by protecting your feelings while remaining open to love.

Setting and maintaining boundaries

One of the most important skills to develop when it comes to relationships is setting boundaries. Many people are afraid of setting boundaries because they fear they will be pushing love and relationships away. But boundaries are simply healthy limits, helping us to define who we are and providing clarity on what we feel comfortable with, both for ourselves and others.

For emotionally sensitive people, boundaries are particularly important because we absorb so much of what other people are feeling and often feel compelled to help them. Dr Judith Orloff refers to HSPs as emotional empaths, and suggests that many have difficulty keeping relationships because they fail to articulate their needs. Sensitive people need a lot of quiet time to themselves, as well as physical and emotional space in order to relax and recover from the constant stimulation of other people's energy, which can be a challenge in a relationship, as the sensitive person can easily feel crowded or overwhelmed and the partner can find it difficult to understand. If the feelings around them are positive, sensitive people will reflect the love and kindness they absorb. But if others' feelings are hostile, angry, fearful, aggressive or any other form of negative energy, sensitive people will also absorb these feelings and quickly become drained and exhausted, anxious, depressed and experience an array of mental and physical symptoms, often leaving them without the strength to separate themselves from the negative feelings or from the negative person. Defining and expressing your mutual needs, and setting appropriate boundaries, is essential.

Boundaries involve two steps: setting them and enforcing them. Relationships test our boundaries, so it's important to know where to draw the line. It can be difficult to know when to say yes and when to say no, especially when you are emotionally involved with someone and you are sensitive enough to feel their feelings. Saying no can feel selfish, like a betrayal. But it isn't. Saying no is an important part of looking after yourself. In the words of boundaries experts Dr Henry Cloud and Dr John Townsend, 'separating ourselves protects love, because we are taking a stand against things that destroy love'.

While it is essential to say no to what feels wrong, it is just as important to say yes to support from others, especially when you are in the process of trying to establish your boundaries. We all need help and we are all part of a larger community that works when it works together. Don't be afraid to ask for help and lean on others for support.

The key to knowing when to draw a boundary line is to listen to your own feelings. They are there to help you. If you feel afraid, angry, upset, confused or any other uncomfortable feeling, it's best to say no and take a step back. Trust your own feelings and your instincts, even when someone is trying to convince you that everything is all right. If it feels bad or wrong *to* you, it is bad or wrong *for* you. That's all the proof you need.

When you know yourself and you know what you need, setting clear boundaries becomes easier. Listening to your own feelings will guide you. You need to express your needs and your boundaries to others, and respect their boundaries as well. The difficulty often comes when someone crosses your boundary and you feel victimized, invaded, insulted and angry. Sometimes people will test your boundaries just to see if you really mean what you say. You want to say something, but you don't know what to say and perhaps you are afraid that you will lose that person if you do. But mindful relationships do not act in fear. They act out of love. And real love accepts your limits and boundaries and your needs with respect.

If someone crosses your boundary line it's important to enforce it. Let the person know she has crossed a boundary. She may apologize and admit to making a mistake, for which you can forgive her. Or if she continually crosses your boundary, or becomes angry or ignores you, she is showing a clear lack of respect for your needs, in which case you may need to reconsider the relationship. To enforce your boundaries there need to be consequences. Talk to the other person, tell her your needs and your concerns and then if she ignores them you can tell her what the consequences will be.

Kelly began to set boundaries for herself because she was unhappy in her relationships. She realized she was allowing men to control her because she believed she should sacrifice herself for others. Recognizing that that was no longer true for her, she started telling the man she was dating that she wouldn't tidy up the house for him when she came to visit. She explained that if he continued to tell her to do it, she wouldn't come to visit any more. He stopped calling her. Eventually she met someone else and tried again. He was the same kind of controlling person, and when she asserted her boundaries and told him what she wasn't comfortable with, he tried to talk her out of it. He bought her chocolates and told her she would do it if she really loved him. She wanted to make him happy and saying no felt wrong; it felt selfish and she questioned whether she was really doing the right thing. But when she started letting herself be controlled again she noticed how depressed she felt and then she knew it wasn't right. So she decided to end the relationship. Eventually, she started meeting men who weren't controlling and who respected her. Because she had enforced her boundaries, she was no longer attractive to controlling men.

Protecting yourself from negative feelings

While other people's behaviour can make relationships a challenge, their feelings and the feelings they generate in you can become overwhelming as well, especially for sensitive types. Sensitive people, such as those prone to fear and anxiety, often absorb the feelings of other people and take them on as their own. Growing up as a sensitive child often meant not only feeling the emotions of your parents and siblings, but wanting to do something about it. Children want to protect their parents from suffering so that they will be happy and then the child will be happy. But it is an exhausting, debilitating and ultimately fruitless job because you cannot make anyone else happy. Psychologist Wendy Gillissen advises sensitive people to remember one important fact when it comes to relationships: just because you can sense other people's feelings doesn't mean you are responsible for them. This is key to becoming free from the exhaustion and fear generated by other people. You are not responsible for other people's feelings. You are not responsible for other people. It can be very hard to accept that people have to make mistakes and learn on their own, especially when it's someone you care about and you can see them struggling or suffering with their own feelings. But to step in and take on those feelings for them and to take on the responsibility of dealing with them would take away the opportunity for them to grow. And that is just what we all need to do, each in our own way, on our own, according to the lessons we each need to learn.

Mindfulness allows you to release any feelings of obligation towards others by making you aware of which feelings belong to you and which feelings belong to others. The following simple exercise will allow you to distinguish between your feelings and someone else's and free you from becoming engulfed by other people's energy:

- Give yourself a moment of quiet whenever you are feeling upset, overwhelmed or aware of uncomfortable feelings. Find a solitary space, such as a quiet room, a garden or even the washroom at work.
- Take a few deep breaths. Then ask yourself, 'What is this emotion that I'm feeling?' Try not to think about it, just listen and it will come to you. It may come as words or a voice or an image.
- When you know what you are feeling, ask yourself, 'Who do these feelings belong to?' Again, just listen and the person will come to you. If the feelings are yours then you can decide what to do. For example, if you are experiencing anxiety and you find that the feelings are actually fear, you can ask yourself why you are feeling that way. You will know. Trust yourself. It can be incredibly empowering to discover and accept your own emotions.
- If you ask yourself who the feelings belong to and your boss's face comes to mind, or your mother's or your ex-boyfriend's, then take a deep breath and, as you exhale, let the feelings go. Say to yourself, 'These feelings do not belong to me. I am not responsible for them.' Focus on your own breathing and let those feelings go.

Looking after your emotions is as important as looking after your physical needs for food, water and sleep. You will feel calmer, safer, stronger and more confident when you learn to honour your own needs for peace and quiet throughout the day. Pay attention to what stresses or upsets you and give yourself permission to get what you need. Don't feel guilty about looking after yourself. It's okay. Taking care of yourself is your first priority. Once you are in a position of calm and happiness you can then start helping others, and you will bring your love and joy with you.

Here are a few ways to find some peace from negative emotions:

- Give yourself some quiet time alone throughout the day. Breathe. Stretch. Take a walk.
- Meditate. When you are feeling overwhelmed, take a moment to centre your energy and move the focus away from others.
- Release the negative feelings by writing in your journal.
- Honour your needs:
  - Say no to requests that are too much for you.
  - Limit the time you spend in groups and bring your own transportation so you can leave when you need to.
  - Eat high-protein meals frequently and mindfully, to keep you grounded.
  - Find a private space at home to retreat to.

Dealing with difficult people

Unfortunately, there are many selfish people in the world who will take advantage of your need for love and will use your dependence on them to fuel their own selfish needs. Learn to recognize people who can bring you down. People who are particularly difficult include the criticizer, the victim, the narcissist and the controller. Judith Orloff terms these people 'emotional vampires'. When you know how to recognize these types of people you can protect yourself against them, including removing yourself from their presence. Avoiding these kinds of people means that you stop relying on others to make you feel loved and start relying on yourself. The need for other people's approval is the fear-based way of trying to be loved. Approving of yourself is the mindful way. Give yourself what you are looking for and you will not only feel better about yourself, you will start attracting people like you – people who are kind, compassionate, loving and healthy.

Most of us have had painful experiences with difficult people, but sensitive people not only seem to attract challenging types more often, they are also most affected by it. By recognizing the often invisible but potent attraction between emotionally sensitive people and more aggressive or negative types, you can find the tools not only to recover from your trying experiences, but the knowledge and strength to avoid them in the future.

One of the most common and most challenging types of relationship is with narcissists. Narcissists are people who lack empathy, possess a grandiose sense of self-importance and a need for admiration and attention. They do not care about the feelings or needs of other people, except in the way that others can fulfil their own needs, because they believe they are special and are entitled to special treatment. They often see people simply as tools, including their own family members and their own children.

Narcissists are particularly attracted to sensitive people because they can sense their empathy, compassion and their deep concern for others. Narcissists will essentially feed off the kindness of others like emotional vampires until the sensitive person is left emotionally drained and powerless. Unfortunately, narcissism is rarely 'cured', partially because narcissists don't think there's anything wrong with them. Any kind of relationship with a narcissist is going to be difficult and emotionally painful. The best way to deal with narcissists is to avoid them as much as possible. If you are involved with a narcissist that you cannot avoid, here are some tips for coping:

Learn to recognize the traits of a narcissist   Beware of people who seem a little too preoccupied with their appearance, their status and what people think of them. Recognize that you, as an HSP, are vulnerable to them.

Lower your expectations   Narcissists can be extremely charming, intelligent and fun. But they will never give you what you need. They will use any means, including deception, passive–aggression, control tactics and manipulation to get what they want.

Don't seek their approval   Narcissists will always use you to boost their own ego and make your sense of self-worth dependent on them. Learn to feel good about yourself by yourself.

Communicate effectively   Openness and honesty do not work with narcissists because they don't care about your feelings. Angry demands do not work either. If you must interact, tell them how they will benefit to get what you want.

Walk away   If you start feeling drained in someone's company, politely excuse yourself and move at least 20 feet away. If you feel immediate relief, you will know this person is someone for you to avoid.

Keeping fear in its place: nurturing healthy relationships

We are all affected by other people's feelings and we often feel the urge to help others when they are distressed, but then feel overwhelmed by their feelings. We also find ourselves acting defensively towards others or blaming them for our unpleasant feelings. But anger, denial, blame and withdrawal only exacerbate the negative feelings in our relationships and make us feel lonely, rejected or guilty. By becoming aware of why we argue and why we blame our partner, however, we can create relationships based on love and trust instead of fear.

Your thoughts and the negative beliefs behind them trigger the survival response that creates feelings of fear, and the reaction to fear is often blame, denial, anger, avoidance or defensiveness, all of which give temporary relief from the fear, but ultimately give your fear more power and your relationship less trust.

We should not be simply surviving in relationships, but thriving. They are meant to bring out the best in us and to make us feel loved and cherished. But the best relationships also allow us to be vulnerable enough not only to give and accept love, but to face the negative beliefs that have long been holding us back. It's in relationships that these beliefs most often rise to the surface of our awareness. Frightening though they may be, the key is not to suppress these thoughts and feelings, or to blame the other person, but to accept them and deal with them head on.

A healthy relationship will not only trigger your negative beliefs, but provide you with the perfect opportunity and support you need to face them and ultimately let them go. While we have to deal with our own fears ourselves, we can also turn to others for help. We are all part of a larger community and other people are there to help us and guide us and offer a sympathetic ear or perhaps a shoulder to lean on. You still have to do the work yourself, but sharing your fears with someone trustworthy can give you the strength, support, reassurance and grounding you need to let go of your limiting beliefs and move forward, while creating a nurturing and trusting relationship with that person in the process.

Many of us feel the urge to walk or run away from relationships when they become challenging. When the romantic bliss of the first few months of a relationship seem to have worn off and you begin to experience misunderstandings and arguments in what was previously a happy and loving partnership, it's easy to think that the relationship is doomed or that you are simply incompatible. But it's often the very moment when you are beginning to feel vulnerable with someone, when are you letting your guard down and developing trust for them, that your fears rise to the surface, as do those of your partner. When we respond to our fears and insecurities with defensiveness, blame and anger, our relationships suffer.

The reality is that these kinds of arguments are indications of personal growth. In his book *Getting the Love You Want*, Dr Harville Hendrix asserts that 'in most interactions with your spouse, you are actually safer when you lower your defences than when you keep them engaged, because your partner becomes an ally, not an enemy'.

Part of a love relationship's purpose is to heal childhood wounds. It's an environment in which your subconscious mind feels comfortable and safe enough to release your fears into your conscious mind and into your thoughts. It's your reaction to those thoughts that causes the arguments, however, not the other person. Even though you know it's someone you care about, your survival instinct kicks in and you react as if you are under attack, and attack or flee in return. Of course people will always make mistakes and do or say hurtful things, and you may find yourself irritated with some aspects of a person's personality as you discover more about him or her. But it's essential to look inward and ask yourself what you are afraid of when you are blaming the other person. Why are you so angry? There is a reason why someone else's behaviour is triggering such an emotional response in you. And it's usually not because what they are doing is so awful but because it reminds you of some similar event that hurt you in the past.

Kelly had always been attracted to controlling men because they subconsciously reminded her of her father. She didn't like to be controlled, but it was familiar to her. Nevertheless, she always found herself arguing with her boyfriends when they became controlling because their behaviour triggered a fear response in her. She was afraid she was going to be controlled by a bully the way she was by her father and she feared feeling hurt. The controlling men didn't like to argue with her because they feared losing their control over her, and so the relationships ended. She had tried to avoid the pain of being controlled by blaming the men she dated, while they in turn became angry and defensive. She realized that her relationship problems originated from her own fears and her attempts to cope with those fears through blame and avoidance. When she stopped blaming others, and instead talked with her new boyfriend about how some of his behaviour triggered her own feelings of fear, their arguments began to turn into discussions. He no longer felt attacked and she no longer felt afraid. She felt supported and understood. And by allowing herself to be vulnerable with her fears with someone she trusted, Kelly gained the confidence to banish her fears and build a relationship based on mutual respect.

The amazingly healing thing about vulnerability and trust in intimate relationships is that what one partner needs the most is what the other partner is often least able to give. For example, Kelly needs to feel that her needs count as much as anyone else's, and yet she finds partners who don't respect her needs. But that is also the exact issue where her partner needs to grow. So by giving what Kelly needs, which in this case is not to be controlled, her partner grows and learns to be in a relationship without being controlling and so he gains confidence in himself as well.

Here are some further suggestions for how to face the fears that are affecting your relationship and nurture yourself as well as your partner:

- When you hear yourself becoming angry, defensive or blaming, stop and ask yourself what you are afraid of. Are you afraid of rejection, abandonment, or being controlled?
- Talk to your partner. Tell him or her that you are upset because you are feeling fear and explain those fears.
- Listen to your partner. Your partner has his or her own fears as well and they need to be heard without judgement, criticism or trying to minimize or fix them. Just listen and acknowledge how he or she is feeling.
- Recognize that you will trigger fears in each other. For example, Brian expressed his fear that he was not good enough for anyone, which triggered his wife's fear that he was going to leave her. But accepting your fears together means you can help each other face them.
- Accept that overcoming your fears will take time and practice. Fears won't disappear overnight. They are caused by an instinct for survival whenever you feel that you might get hurt. You might tell

your partner that there's no real reason for her to fear abandonment, but you cannot expect her to simply 'get over it' because it makes sense. Instead, offer patience and reassurance and allow both of you time to heal.

Relationships, especially love relationships, can be conflicted and painful, giving rise to our deepest fears. They make us want to run and hide or fight back, lashing out at the person who appears to be the source of so much pain. But the pain and the fear came from a long-ago place, before you were able to look after yourself. The relationships you have with others now are within your control. You can meet your needs for love and commitment, for approval and respect and loyalty, and meet those of your partner. But it means standing in the face of fear and acknowledging its presence head on. It means not running from your feelings, not blaming your partner, but working together to heal wounds. We need relationships because they connect us to who we really are, and because they give us not only the joys of love but the strength to be ourselves.

12

Creativity, work and dreams

The work you do should be a reflection of you, enabling you to use your passions, your creativity and talents, your skills and interests in a way that creates success, helps others and fills you with a sense of purpose and fulfilment. Working in the wrong job, feeling that your dreams are stifled or not knowing what your real dreams are, can feel so wrong that it drains the spirit out of you, leaving you without the energy to take another step towards what you really want. They are also indications of fear. Your fear works against you, stopping you from leaving the job you hate and fulfilling your own desires. The good news is that you don't have to wait for someone else to make your dreams come true. You can do something about it.

In this chapter, we'll look at how fear affects our work and dreams, the role of creativity in our lives, and the ways in which we sabotage our own success by succumbing to the power of fear. Fear isn't necessarily going to disappear, but you can ensure that it doesn't control your life or your decisions. When it comes to your choices regarding your work, and whether you consider that work your career, your calling or your dream, it is important that you make those choices consciously without being controlled by fear, because what you do in life and how you use your passion not only reflects who you are and the way you see yourself, but it can fill you up in a way nothing else can.

How we sabotage our success

Fear can create chains around us, shackling us to a job, a situation or a belief that makes it feel like we will be tethered to this unhappy existence forever. While we may not like the situation we are in, we often sabotage our own happiness by talking ourselves out of change because of our own fears.

Fear has many faces and takes many forms, and it's different for everyone. But when it comes to our working lives, many of us recognize the familiar face of the fear of rejection and the fear of failure. We can also fear taking a risk, we can fear change, we can fear that our dreams are too outrageous and therefore impossible. We can simply fear that what we want to do will be too hard or too much work. The fear of what others think can also be frightening, whether we are afraid that someone might think what we want to do is foolish or inappropriate or impossible.

Sometimes the fear is based not on other people's opinions but our own. We can feel that we are not doing a good job or that we are somehow not smart enough, good enough or creative enough to go for our dreams. But the way we feel about ourselves has a huge effect on whether we choose to go for those dreams or not. Making dreams come true is not about how clever or talented you are, but whether or not you believe you can do it. You need to be willing to make mistakes and face challenges, to take risks and persevere despite criticism from others.

All these fears can lead us to give up on the things we want the most, and to use distractions as a way of avoiding dealing with our own pain. In the cycle of avoidance we can keep fear at arm's length by busying ourselves with other tasks, like watching TV, surfing the Internet, shopping or socializing, so that we never have to think about what is really holding us back.

Likewise, we can avoid facing our own fears by pointing the finger at a lack of money or lack of time so that we don't have to look at ourselves as the real reason we are not getting what we want. But these are just excuses. And by blaming time or money or other people for our lives, we remain where we started – unhappy and frustrated and unfulfilled.

While these fears are common, all of them have the result of making you stop in your tracks and settle for what you have instead of fighting for what you want. Standing up to your own fears can feel like you are wrestling with your jailer in a dark cell as you struggle to pull the shackles from your ankles. But the alternative is to sit down and do nothing, letting life pass you by and watching your own dreams die, and pieces of yourself with them.

Mindfulness allows you to face your fear, your jailer, and recognize him for what he is, a tired old nag who is trying to control you by putting negative thoughts in your head. Seeing fear for what it is can release those shackles and give you the first step towards freedom. Instead of avoiding our painful feelings of self-doubt, self-criticism and fear, we need to face them, accept them and push through them so that they no longer control us.

Discover your calling

One of the most important tools you need to help you face your fear is knowing what you want. We discussed the ways in which you can unravel your personality in Chapter 5. But what about your career? How do your personality and your individual needs affect your career choices? And how do your career choices affect you?

Moving fearlessly towards your dreams can be difficult when you are not sure which direction you want to move towards. Our fears can cloud our vision, making it difficult to see past the self-doubt and feelings of inadequacy or criticism from others. One way to clear through that haze of confusion is to think back to a time before the influence of fear set in. Most of our dreams and passions, interests and talents were in plain sight when we were growing up, before we listened to the opinions of others and before we started censoring ourselves.

What did you like to do when you were a child? Did you spend all your free time drawing or dancing or building model airplanes? Or perhaps you loved organizing games and activities for all the neighbourhood children. While it may seem like just child's play, the things we did when we were young are often the things that we still like to do, but we have simply forgotten about them, dismissed them as 'childish' or let someone talk us out of it. Think back to what you liked to do, look at old photos and toy collections and you will see your true passions emerge. You can even try out your old stuff again, just for fun. Get out your painting-by-numbers set or your dolls and see what happens. Even as adults we need to play to give ourselves a break from the duties and responsibilities of life and to let our creativity express itself. Look at the way children play. There is no fear, no questioning their own motives or behaviour. There is only living in the moment, and living in joy. Play gives you that freedom.

Even as an adult, take note of what excites you now. Do you drag yourself through your day at work yet find yourself talking excitedly to a friend about your story ideas or doodling new house designs instead of writing shopping lists? Learn to become aware of where you are spending your time and how it makes you feel. Your calling could be hiding just under that pile of work on your desk, in the garden shed or in your recipe box. Don't dismiss things just because they seem commonplace or dull. There is magic in everyday moments.

If you have discovered your Myers–Briggs personality type or read David Keirsey's *Please Understand Me II*, then you will find a further valuable source of information on careers based on your personality type. The key is doing something that works for the kind of person that you are. The more you understand who you are and what you need, the easier it will be to narrow down your options to what really feels right.

Once you have an idea of what you might like to do, talk to people in careers you are interested in and ask them about their work. Most people are happy to talk to you about their jobs and their interests and may even give you some tips for getting started.

> Anne worked in an advertising agency, but she had never felt happy there. In fact, just the thought of completing spreadsheets or attending meetings filled her with anxiety and dread. At home, however, she relaxed when she could spend some time drawing with her children and reading them stories. She had always thought that she simply enjoyed being a parent. But after talking to friends, who encouraged her to take her drawing seriously, she started looking into her past and doing some reading. She had always loved creating stories and painting as a girl. She had just never thought of it as a career. She started taking art classes and wrote down all her ideas until one day she started writing a children's picture book. After creating her own website and posting some of her stories and artwork, she found a publisher for her book.

If you are an HSP you probably feel the need to do something meaningful in your work. It isn't enough just to have a job or even a career. You need to find your calling. What this means is that you are doing something that allows you to express your special gifts and feel appreciated for what you do as well as help others and nurture their growth in a way that doesn't drain you.

Releasing your creativity

We all have the ability to be creative. Creativity allows you to express your thoughts and feelings and beliefs as well as release stress and find a powerful outlet for the overwhelming energy you absorb around you as a sensitive person. Without releasing that energy, we can easily become not only overwhelmed ourselves but exhausted, frustrated, depressed and subject to any number of ailments, both physical and mental. But that urge to create can easily become stifled by our own fears. Whether your creativity becomes a vocation or simply a way of expressing who you are, it is an important part of your health and happiness. So how do you find your creative side and let it out? And how do you keep it coming?

Many people believe that if they write a bestseller or star in a film or somehow become famous that they will no longer feel afraid of failure or criticism or self-doubt, because they will have found success. But if you are doing something creative to become rich or famous, then you still will not escape your own fears because you are constantly seeking external gratification instead of internal fulfilment. Creative pursuits feel good because they hold meaning for you. If they don't, you will feel empty, and so will the audience you are trying to connect with. People appreciate passion and it shows in the work that you do. The best part of any creative enterprise is not the money or the fame or even the recognition, but the moment you are doing it, sitting at your desk, huddled at the kitchen table at 3 a.m., where there is just you and your connection to something deeper. That is mindfulness.

But fear can prevent us from getting to that connected place. Perhaps you feel that you are not one of those creative types or that if you try you are going to fail. Perhaps you feel that your work isn't good enough. Perhaps you are waiting for genius to strike. The truth is that art comes through hard work and perseverance and practice. A few people have been able to create masterpieces seemingly without trying but, for most of us, creativity is a process. But that doesn't mean it's any less worthy. Art in any form can be intimidating because it appears to be perfect. But writers, musicians, artists and dancers all have to practise and revise their work to get it just right. And they practise every day, whether they feel inspired or not. Sometimes just showing up at the same time every day, and thinking of yourself as a creative person, is enough to get your creative juices flowing. Creativity is an amazing way of getting in touch with your own fears and thoughts and beliefs as well, because it comes from your subconscious mind. Thinking about your responsibilities and worries keeps you in your conscious mind. When you stop thinking and let your instincts take over, your creative thoughts step forward.

Showing up also requires you to slow down. Our lives can be so busy and hectic that we never have the mental space to allow creative thoughts to emerge. When you are tired, creativity is the first thing to go because it is energy. And when your mind is consumed with thoughts of tonight's dinner or next week's meeting or what your in-laws really think of you, the creativity welling up inside you remains locked away. Relaxation opens the door. A relaxed mind is a creative mind. To find the key to that door, look for ways to relax. Many sensitive people find spending time in nature or with animals to be very soothing. Set aside a special time each day just for being creative, and then light a few candles and put on some music and take a deep breath and focus on the present moment. It doesn't matter what you create or what anyone thinks of your work. Don't even worry about what you think of your work. You are probably your own worst critic.

Mindful creativity means that you stop censoring your own creative energy by acknowledging and then letting go of your thoughts and focusing on the moment. When we allow ourselves to slow down and take the time to do something for ourselves, we often initially find our minds swimming with to-do lists and worries, with fears that we don't have time for our own needs, fears that we are being selfish or ridiculous or shameful, or fears that our creative work will not be valued because we are not a 'real' artist. You may also become aware that you are avoiding your creative activities when you notice thoughts such as, 'I am scared of starting a painting. I can't do it. I will do the laundry instead.' When you hear these thoughts, you can recognize them as your excuses and complaints and your fears. And then you can decide what to do. What do you really want to do? Painting isn't frightening. Your fear of failure is frightening. If you decide you would rather paint than do laundry, if you would rather become a painter than someone who always wanted to paint, then look at your fear and let it go. Then grab your paintbrushes and let it unfold.

Once you shift the mental chatter away, and give yourself the time to breathe, your creative ideas will begin to appear like blossoms emerging from a patiently tended garden.

How to make dreams a reality

So you have figured out who you are and what you want. You are working on identifying the fears that are holding you back and learning to banish any self-defeating beliefs about yourself. The next step is to move from awareness of your dreams to actually living them. The surprising thing is that you have already done the hard part. Simply knowing what you want and believing that you can do it, in spite of your fears and what anyone else thinks, will automatically set a path for you in the direction you want to go. The next stage is simply to take a step forward.

Act

Thinking about what you want and planning your career and your dream life is like planting the seeds for the garden you want. But to make it grow you have to do more than sit back and wait. You have to act. This is your life. If you want something to happen, you need to do something to make it happen. It can seem overwhelming if you are working in an accounting office but you really want to be leading walking tours through the Himalayas or writing screenplays in Hollywood. The key is to break it all down into small tasks and to do something every day that moves you closer to your goal. When you take a risk, you realize that it was worth it and then you start dreaming bigger and bigger. The biggest risk you can take is to not follow your own dreams.

> Stan had been working for the same company for 10 years and he was bored. He was stuck in a rut and wanted a new challenge. He loved spending time with his friends and colleagues and everyone told him what a great listener he was and how understanding he was with their problems. He began to think about becoming a therapist, and the more he thought about it the more excited he became. Helping other people was something he had always enjoyed, even as a boy. So he started taking action to move closer to his dream job. He read psychology books and started taking a counselling class. And then he discovered, to his surprise, that listening to people talk about their problems left him feeling drained and overwhelmed. It was different from just listening to his friends. It was too much for him. Feeling discouraged, Stan looked for other ways to help people and so he started writing a blog. Soon, people began commenting on his posts, telling him how helpful he was. Stan had discovered that although he loved people he was also a very sensitive person, and that other people's feelings easily overwhelmed him. But when he wrote about issues that concerned people, he could help them without becoming overwhelmed. It wasn't long before Stan started writing for magazines and getting paid for doing what he loved.

One of the advantages of being a sensitive person is that you have a wellspring of energy within you that you can use to drive your ambitions. Drive or motivation is what gets you off the sofa and sitting at your desk, writing that novel, designing furniture or creating a business plan. Sensitive people are often anxious people because they are constantly absorbing energy from people around them. Fear is energy too. It makes your hands shake and your heart pound. This can be overwhelming, and so you can retreat from this anxious energy and hide under the covers or you can channel it into your work, your creative pursuits and your dreams.

Being sensitive also means that you notice things more than other people, providing you with endless sources of inspiration. Instead of trying to keep sensory and emotional stimulation at bay because it feels like 'too much', put it into your work. Sensitive people also need a lot of quiet time alone, which means that you can think about things you have noticed and absorbed and process things in a creative way. Not only will you find a healthy and calming release for your feelings and your anxieties, you will also be creating something beautiful that will inevitably inspire others.

Ernest Hemingway's advice for aspiring authors who wanted to write novels was simply to write one true sentence. That's all he did. Instead of sitting down to write a novel, he told himself to just write one true thing. When you give yourself little steps to take, the pressure eases and the dream doesn't seem so intimidating or impossible. You can write just one true sentence. You can draw an apple. You can send one email. It doesn't have to be right or perfect but just true and genuine. Don't criticize or edit yourself. Chances are, you will look up to find you have written a whole page, designed a new pattern or created an original idea. When you do things as if no one were watching, as if no one will ever know, you can create amazing things.

Cope

While you are taking steps to move your life in a new direction you can still become discouraged, depressed or overwhelmed by the reality of your daily life. It's important to take care of yourself and if you are an HSP you have special needs for adequate sleep, rest, relaxation and nourishment, in addition to the need to spend enough time alone to recharge your batteries and express your creative energy.

While you are nurturing your dreams one step at a time, here are some tips for coping with the day job that will allow you to live the life you want and still pay the bills:

Prioritize your work Make to-do lists and schedule enough time to complete each task.

Plan ahead Write due dates on your calendar and get started on big projects as early as you can to avoid a last-minute panic.

Anticipate problems Try to foresee obstacles and work to deal with them at the beginning.

Set boundaries Know your limits and ask for help or delegate tasks if you need to.

Communicate Talk to your supervisor if you run into difficulties and be up-front and open about problems. Ask for what you need. A lot of work stress is generated by lack of communication.

Organize Keep your desk clear and your papers filed so you don't waste time looking for things. Clutter can make you feel stressed too, so keep it under control.

Avoid negative people If there are people at work who drain your energy or you feel bad around, try to avoid dealing with them.

Take breaks A walk outside or a few minutes of breathing mindfully can relax you.

Use employer resources Many companies offer an employee assistance programme that includes gym discounts, classes and counselling.

Be open to possibilities

Finding a comfortable balance between supporting yourself financially and supporting yourself spiritually comes down to knowing and valuing your unique traits and creating the work that's right for you. For example, many HSPs are sensitive to the feelings of others. This is often a detriment in an office environment, where you end up absorbing everyone else's work. But there are jobs where that kind of empathy would be a great asset, such as counselling, teaching, health care and veterinary medicine. Are you creative? Perhaps you love gardening. And you are inspired by helping others. Put all those skills and interests together and you could be developing outdoor special needs programmes or teaching gardening classes to adults or perhaps writing a gardening book for children.

Don't try to squeeze yourself into a work role. Instead, carve out a role that fits you, based on your own unique talents, interests, abilities and temperament. One of the best options for sensitive or anxious people is self-employment, because it allows you to do the work that you want to do and in the way you like to do it. Not everyone functions well in an office environment full of noise and bright lights and lots of other people.

> Brian had a demanding job where he was struggling to cope with stress as well as trying to cope with the demands of his family. He decided to start his own business and become self-employed. He finds the rewards of doing work he loves and fulfilling his purpose are life-changing, even with the challenges of finding new clients and doing the administrative work himself.

When you follow the path that is right for you you can focus on the end goal. Let go of the 'how' and focus on the 'what'. The desire to make things happen a certain way is often what causes fear and despair and makes people want to give up. Things may not be happening the way they wanted or it may appear as though nothing is happening at all, when in fact things are simply taking a different route that we cannot see.

> Kelly, who had suffered as a child with an alcoholic father and had been in a series of unhappy relationships with alcoholics, couldn't understand why life seemed so cruel and unfair. She was bored at work and her life felt meaningless. But as she began to understand herself and her fears better, she learned more about alcoholism and how it affects people. She wanted to study but she didn't know how she could afford it until she discovered a free mentoring scheme that provided counsellor training, enabling her to use her difficult experiences to help others. She never planned to be a counsellor but she felt driven to help others who had gone through the same things she had, and she found that kind of work infinitely rewarding.

Sometimes, the best thing we can do to alleviate our fears is to do the things that we like to do best. And these are often the very things that are causing us to feel fear. We love drawing or writing poetry, but we fear that our work is not good enough and we'll be ridiculed. Spending time doing those things, however, will not only improve your skills and your chances of success, but fill your soul and your heart with the sense of fullness and completion that you have been looking for. You don't have to go out looking for your dreams. They are all there inside you, waiting to be released.

References

Introduction

Ankrom, Sheryl. 'What's the difference between fear and anxiety?'. About.com, May 2009. <http://panicdisorder.about.com/od/understandingpanic/a/fearandanxiety.htm>.

Hatloy, Inger. *Understand Anxiety and Panic Attacks*. Mind, London, 2012.

Kabat-Zinn, J. *Full Catastrophe Living: Using the Wisdom of your Mind to Face Stress, Pain and Illness*. Dell Publishing, New York, 1990.

Kabat-Zinn, J. *Mindfulness for Beginners*. Sounds True, Louisville, CO, 2006.

Kaplan, Harold I. and Sadock, Benjamin J. *Synopsis of Psychiatry*, 8th ed. Williams & Wilkins, Baltimore, 1998.

Mayo Clinic. 'Anxiety'. <www.mayoclinic.com/health/anxiety/DS01187/DSECTION=risk-factors>.

Mental Health Foundation. 'Fear and anxiety'. <www.mentalhealth.org.uk/help-information/mental-health-a-z/F/fear-anxiety/>.

Mind. 'Anxiety and panic attacks'. <www.mind.org.uk/mental_health_a-z/8001_understanding_anxiety_and_panic_attacks>.

1 Causes of fear and anxiety

Henig, Robin Marantz. 'Understanding the anxious mind'. *New York Times*, September 2009. <www.nytimes.com/2009/10/04/magazine/04anxiety-t.html?pagewanted=all&_r=0>.

Kagan, J. *Galen's Prophecy: Temperament in Human Nature*. Westview Press, Boulder, CO, 1997.

Miller, Dale T. and McFarland, Cathy. 'Pluralistic ignorance: When similarity is interpreted as dissimilarity'. *Journal of Personality and Social Psychology*, 1987; 53(2): 298–305.

Montag, C., Buckholtz, J. W., Hartmann, P. *et al*. 'COMT genetic variation affects fear processing: Psychophysiological evidence'. *Behavioral Neuroscience*, 2008; 122(4): 901–9.

Rafaeli, Eshkol, Bernstein, David P. and Young, Jeffrey. *Schema Therapy*. Guilford Press, New York, 2006.

Shumyatsky, G. P., Malleret, G., Shin, R. M. *et al*. 'Stathmin, a gene enriched in lateral nucleus of amygdala, controls both learned and innate fear'. *Cell*, 2005; 123: 697–709.

Sichel, Mark. 'Upload character when you're hard-wired to worry'. *Psychology Today*, October 2009. <www.psychologytoday.com/blog/the-therapist-is-in/200910/upload-character-when-youre-hard-wired-worry>.

2 Where fear emerges

Bowlby, J. *Separation: Anxiety and Anger: Attachment and Loss*, Vol. 2. Random House, New York, 1998.

Lederbogen, F., Kirsch, P., Haddad, L. *et al.* 'City living and urban upbringing affect neural social stress processing in humans'. *Nature*, 2011; 474(7352): 498–501.

Le Sage, B. 'Familiarity principle of attraction', in Reis, H. T. and Sprecher, S. (Eds) *Encyclopedia of Human Relationships*. Sage, New York, 2009.

Magalhaes, A. C., Holmes, K. D., Dale, L. B. *et al.* 'CRF receptor 1 regulates anxiety behavior via sensitization of 5-HT2 receptor signaling'. *Nature Neuroscience*, 2010; 3(5): 622–9.

Michie, S. 'Causes and management of stress at work'. *Occupational and Environmental Medicine*, 2002; 59(1): 67–72.

3 Triggers of anxiety and fear

Anxiety and Depression Association of America. 'Stress and anxiety interfere with sleep'. <www.adaa.org/understanding-anxiety/related-illnesses/other-related-conditions/stress/stress-and-anxiety-interfere>.

Dray, Sarah. 'Foods and activities that make anxiety worse'. Livestrong.com, October 2010. <www.livestrong.com/article/288126-foods-activities-that-make-anxiety-worse/>.

Iliades, Chris. '7 Surprising causes of anxiety'. Everyday Health, August 2011. <www.everydayhealth.com/anxiety-pictures/7-surprising-causes-of-anxiety.aspx#/slide-5>.

Mayo Clinic. 'Anxiety: Lifestyle and home remedies'. <www.mayoclinic.com/health/anxiety/DS01187/DSECTION=lifestyle-and-home-remedies>.

Michie, S. 'Causes and management of stress at work'. *Occupational and Environmental Medicine*, 2002; 59(1): 67–72.

Strine, T. W., Chapman, D. P., Kobau, R. and Balluz, L. 'Associations of self-reported anxiety symptoms with health-related quality of life and health behaviors'. *Social Psychiatry and Psychiatric Epidemiology*, 2005; 40(6): 432–8.

'Walnuts, walnut oil, improve reaction to stress'. *Science Daily*. <www.sciencedaily.com/releases/2010/10/101004101141.htm>

'10 Common ways to trigger an anxiety attack', *The Reality of Anxiety*, July 2007. <www.anxiousnomore.blogspot.co.uk/2007/07/10-most-common-ways-to-trigger-anxiety.html>.

4 Paying attention when your body speaks

Anxiety and Depression Association of America. 'Related illnesses'. <www.adaa.org/understanding-anxiety/related-illnesses>.

Borchard, Therese J. '5 Gifts of being highly sensitive: Interview with Douglas Eby'. *PsychCentral*, March 2010. <http://psychcentral.com/blog/archives/2010/03/28/5-gifts-of-being-highly-sensitive/>.

D'Ascenzo, Lori. 'Emotions and your body'. *Enlightened Feelings*. <www. enlightenedfeelings.com/body.html>.

Dotinga, Randy. 'Study shows how stress triggers immune system'. *USA Today*, January 2012. <http://usatoday30.usatoday.com/news/health/ story/health/story/2012-01-24/Study-shows-how-stress-triggers-immune-system/52764924/1>.

Hay, Louise L. *Heal Your Body*. Hay House, New York, 1984.

Hong, Harry. 'Healing highly sensitive body'. <www.highlysensitivebody. com/highlysensbody.html>.

Janov, A. *Why You Get Sick, How You Get Well*. Dove Books, California, 1996.

Mayo Clinic. 'Anxiety: Causes'. <www.mayoclinic.com/health/anxiety/ DS01187/DSECTION=causes>.

O'Rourke, C. and Walsh, E. *The Highly Sensitive Person: Introductory Guide*. Plum Turtle Coaching, 2012. <www.plumturtle.com/PlumTurtleCoach- ing/Home_files/HSP_Intro_Handbook.pdf>.

Rosengren, A., Hawken, S., Ounpuu, S. *et al.* 'Association of psychosocial risk factors with risk of acute myocardial infarction in 11119 cases and 13648 controls from 52 countries (the INTERHEART study): case-control study'. *Lancet*, 2004; 64(9438): 953–62.

US National Library of Medicine. 'Stress'. <www.nlm.nih.gov/medlineplus/ stress.html>.

WebMD. 'Can excessive worry make me physically ill?' <www.webmd. com/balance/guide/how-worrying-affects-your-body?page=2>.

'Anxiety and physical illness'. *Harvard Women's Health Watch*, July 2008. <www.health.harvard.edu/newsletters/Harvard_Womens_Health_ Watch/2008/July/Anxiety_and_physical_illness>.

'Stress, anxiety can make allergy attacks even more miserable and last longer', *Science Daily*, August 2008. <www.sciencedaily.com/ releases/2008/08/080814154327.htm>.

5 Discover who you really are

Aron, Elaine. 'The benefits of being highly sensitive, for ourselves and our world'. *Comfort Zone Online*, August 2005. <www.hsperson.com/ pages/1Aug05.htm>.

Briggs-Myers, I. and Myers, P. B. *Gifts Differing: Understanding Personality Type*. CPP, Mountain View, CA, 1995.

Cloninger, C. R., Zohar, A. H., Hirschmann, S. and Dahan, D. 'The psycho- logical costs and benefits of being highly persistent: Personality profiles distinguish mood disorders from anxiety disorders'. *Journal of Affective Disorders*, 2012; 136(3): 758–6.

Eby, Douglas. 'High ability, high sensitivity, high anxiety'. *Talent Devel- opment Resources*, July 2010. <http://talentdevelop.com/3594/high- ability-high-sensitivity-high-anxiety/>.

Harrington, R. and Loffredo, D. 'The relationship between life satisfaction, self-consciousness, and the Myers-Briggs Type Inventory dimensions'. *Journal of Psychology*, 2001; 135(4): 439–50.

Henig, R. M. 'Understanding the anxious mind'. *New York Times*, September 2009. <www.nytimes.com/2009/10/04/magazine/04anxiety-t. html?pagewanted=all&_r=0>.

Jung, C. G. *Psychological Types, Collected Works*, Vol. 6. Princeton University Press, Princeton, NJ, 1921.

Larsen, R. J. and Buss, D. M. *Personality Psychology*. McGraw-Hill, New York, 2002.

Leary, M. R. and Buckley, K. E. 'Shyness and the pursuit of social acceptance', in W. R. Crozier (Ed.) *Shyness: Development, Consolidation, and Change*. Routledge, New York, 2000.

Leary, M. R. and Kowalski, R. M. *Social Anxiety*. Guilford Press, New York, 1995.

Lickerman, Alex. 'How to know yourself'. *Psychology Today*, September 2011. <www.psychologytoday.com/blog/happiness-in-world/201109/ how-know-yourself>.

Tieger, P. D. and Barron, B. *The Art of Speed Reading People*. Little, Brown, New York, 1998.

Zeisset, C. *The Art of Dialogue: Exploring Personality Differences for More Effective Communication*. Center for Applications of Psychological Type, Gainesville, FL, 2006.

6 How mindfulness works

Anxiety and Depression Association of America. 'Mind–body practices'. <www.adaa.org/understanding-anxiety/related-illnesses/other-related-conditions/stress/mind-body-practices>.

Brown, R. P., Gerbarg, P. L. and Muskin, P. R. *How to Use Herbs, Nutrients and Yoga in Mental Health Care*. W. W. Norton, New York, 2008.

Buczynski, Ruth. 'Changing the brain in one month flat'. *National Institute for the Clinical Application of Behavioral Medicine*, August 2012. <www. nicabm.com/nicabmblog/changing-the-brain-in-one-month-flat/>.

Center for Spirituality and Healing and the Life Science Foundation of the University of Minnesota. 'Mind–body therapies'. <http://takingcharge. csh.umn.edu/explore-healing-practiceswhat-are-mind-body-therapies>.

Gordon, J. *Comprehensive Cancer Care: Integrating Alternative, Complementary, and Conventional Therapies*. Perseus Publishing, Cambridge, MA, 2000.

Greenberg, Melanie. 'Nine essential qualities of mindfulness'. *Psychology Today*, February 2012. <www.psychologytoday.com/blog/ the-mindful-self-express/201202/nine-essential-qualities-mindfulness>.

Gunaratana, B. H. *Mindfulness in Plain English*. Wisdom Publications, Boston, MA, 1996.

Kabat-Zinn, Jon. 'Mindfulness meditation practice CDs and tapes'. <www.mindfulnesscds.com/faq.html>.

Mental Health Foundation. 'About mindfulness'. <http://bemindful.co.uk/about-mindfulness/>.

Mindfulnet.org. 'The neuroscience of mindfulness'. <www.mindfulnet.org/page25.htm>.

Nhat Hanh, Thich. 'Five steps to mindfulness'. *Mindful*. <www.mindful.org/mindfulness-practice/mindfulness-and-awareness/five-steps-to-mindfulness>.

Schenck, Laura. '8 Basic characteristics of mindfulness'. *Mindfulness Muse*, November 2011. <www.mindfulnessmuse.com/mindfulness/8-basic-characteristics-of-mindfulness>.

Siegel, D. J. *Mindsight: The New Science of Personal Transformation*. Bantam, New York, 2010.

Siegel, D. J. 'The science of mindfulness'. *Mindful*. <www.mindful.org/the-science/medicine/the-science-of-mindfulness>.

Staik, Athena. 'Cultivating a practice of mindful breathing: Its benefits'. *PsychCentral*, October 2011. <http://blogs.psychcentral.com/relationships/2011/10/cultivating-a-practice-of-mindful-breathing-its-benefits-1-of-3/>.

Zeidan, F., Johnson, S. K., Diamond, B. J., David, Z. and Goolkasian, P. 'Mindfulness meditation improves cognition: Evidence of brief mental training'. *Consciousness and Cognition*, 2010; 19(2): 597–605.

7 Developing awareness, facing your feelings

Brown, K. and Ryan, R. M. 'The benefits of being present: Mindfulness and its role in psychological well-being'. *Journal of Personality and Social Psychology*, 2003; 84(4): 822–48.

Duvinsky, J. *How to Lose Control and Gain Emotional Freedom: Embracing the 'Dark' Emotions Through Integrative Mindful Exposure*. CreateSpace Independent Publishing Platform, 2012.

Ekman, P. *Emotions Revealed: Recognizing Faces and Feelings to Improve Communication and Emotional Life*. Henry Holt, New York, 2003.

Ekman, P. (Ed.) *Emotional Awareness: A Conversation between the Dalai Lama and Paul Ekman*. Times Books, New York, 2008.

Farnsworth, J. and Sewell, K. 'Fearing the emotional self'. *Journal of Constructivist Psychology*, 2012; 25(3): 251–68.

Goldstein, Elisha. 'The upside to embracing dark emotions'. *PsychCentral*, September 2012. <http://blogs.psychcentral.com/mindfulness/2012/09/the-upside-to-embracing-dark-emotions/>.

Hart, T. 'Opening the contemplative mind in the classroom'. *Journal of Transformative Education*, 2004; 2(1): 28–46.

Huston, D. 'Waking up to ourselves: The use of mindfulness meditation and emotional intelligence in the teaching of communications', in

Kroll, K. (Ed.) *Contemplative Teaching and Learning: New Directions for Community Colleges*, Issue 151. Wiley, Chichester, 2010. <http://com municatingmindfully.homestead.com/files/Huston_Chapter_Preprint. pdf>.

Kabat-Zinn, J. *Wherever You Go There You Are: Mindfulness Meditation for Everyday Life*. Hyperion, New York, 1994.

Lewis, M., Haviland-Jones, J. M. and Feldman-Barrett, L. (Eds) *Handbook of Emotions*. Guilford Press, New York, 2008.

Mental Health Foundation. 'Mindfulness'. <www.mentalhealth.org.uk/ content/site/help-and-information/mental-health-a-z/27011/32776/ mindfulness>.

MentalHelp.net. 'Describing fear may regulate emotional aspects of fear'. <www.mentalhelp.net/poc/view_doc.php?type=news&id=149262&cn =1-Mental>.

Nielsen, L. and Kaszniak, A. W. 'Awareness of subtle emotional feelings: A comparison of long-term meditators and non-meditators'. *Emotion*, 2006; 6(3): 392–405.

Tartakovsky, Margarita. 'Find stress relief by spotting your emotional needs'. *PsychCentral*, July 2012. <http://psychcentral.com/ blog/archives/2012/07/27/find-stress-relief-by-spotting-your-emotional-needs/>.

8 Mindful eating, mindful walking

Albers, S. *Eating Mindfully: How to End Mindless Eating and Enjoy a Balanced Relationship with Food*. New Harbinger Publications, Oakland, CA, 2012.

Andrade, A., Greene, G. W. and Melanson, K. J. 'Eating slowly led to decreases in energy intake within meals in healthy women'. *Journal of the American Dietetic Association*, 2008; 108(7): 1186–91.

Chozen Bays, J. *Mindful Eating: A Guide to Rediscovering a Healthy and Joyful Relationship with Food*. Shambhala Publishing, Boston, MA, 2009.

Chozen Bays, J. 'Mindful eating'. *Psychology Today*, February 2009. <www. psychologytoday.com/blog/mindful-eating/200902/mindful-eating>.

Full Spectrum Coaching and Consulting Services. 'Exploring the wisdom of the labyrinth'. <www.full-spectrum.ca/exploring-the-wisdom-of-the-labyrinth/?doing_wp_cron=1362917778>.

Gallagher, James. 'Processed meat "early death" link'. *BBC News*. <www. bbc.co.uk/news/health-21682779>.

Janson, M. 'The No-Diet diet'. *Family Circle*, April 2008.

MacDonald, A. 'Why eating slowly may help you feel full faster'. *Harvard Health Blog*, October 2010. <www.health.harvard.edu/blog/ why-eating-slowly-may-help-you-feel-full-faster-20101019605>.

Nhat Hahn, Thich. *Peace Is Every Step: The Path of Mindfulness in Everyday Life*. Bantam, New York, 1992.

Otto, M. W. and Smits, J. A. J. *Exercise for Mood and Anxiety: Proven Strategies for Overcoming Depression and Enhancing Well-Being.* Oxford University Press, New York, 2011.

Schiedel, Bonnie. 'Mindful walking: Could it help you?'. *Best Health*, September 2008. <www.besthealthmag.ca/embrace-life/wellness/mindful-walking-could-it-help-you>.

Stewart, C. 'Eat meals slowly: It's worth the time!' *Penn Metabolic and Bariatric Surgery Update*, April 2011. <http://penn-bariatric-weight-loss-surgery.blogspot.co.uk/2011/04/eat-meals-slowly-its-worth-time.html

The Center for Mindful Eating. <www.tcme.org/>.

Weir, Kirsten. 'The exercise effect'. *Monitor on Psychology*, 2011; 42(11): 48. <www.apa.org/monitor/2011/12/exercise.aspx>.

Weisman, A. and Smith, J. *The Beginner's Guide to Insight Meditation.* Wisdom Publications, Somerville, MA, 2010.

Wise, Jeff. 'Nine secrets of courage from "Extreme Fear"'. *Psychology Today*, February 2011. <www.psychologytoday.com/collections/201211/wired-worry/nine-secrets-courage>.

'A path of healing and focus'. <www.thelabyrinthladies.com/7.html>.

'Stomach hormone ghrelin increases desire for high-calorie foods'. Presented by T. Goldstone at The Endocrine Society's 92nd Annual Meeting, San Diego, June 2010. <www.endo-society.org/media/press/2010/StomachHormoneGhrelin.cfm>

9 Meditation and yoga

American Psychological Association. 'What are the benefits of mindfulness'. <www.apa.org/monitor/2012/07-08/ce-corner.aspx>.

Grabovac, A. 'What is mindfulness?'. *Mindfulness Matters.* <www.mindfulness-matters.org/what-is-mindfulness/>

Holzel, B., Lazar, S., Gard, T. *et al.* 'How does mindfulness meditation work? Proposing mechanisms of action from a conceptual and neural perspective'. *Perspectives on Psychological Science*, 2011; 6(6): 537–59.

Huston, D. 'Waking up to ourselves: The use of mindfulness meditation and emotional intelligence in the teaching of communications', in Kroll, K. (Ed.) *Contemplative Teaching and Learning: New Directions for Community Colleges*, Issue 151. Wiley, Chichester, 2010. <http://communicating-mindfully.homestead.com/files/Huston_Chapter_Preprint.pdf>.

Jorgensen Smith, Therese. '15 Minute yoga routine'. *Share Guide.* <www.shareguide.com/yoga15.html>.

Mindful. 'Body and mind integration'. <www.mindful.org/mindfulness-practice/mindfulness-and-awareness/body-and-mind-integration>.

Mindful. 'Meditation: Getting started'. <www.mindful.org/Meditation%20in%20Action/getting-started-with-formal-practice>.

Sakyong Mipham Rinpoche. 'How to do mindfulness meditation'. *Shambhala Sun.* <www.shambhalasun.com/index.php?option=content&task=view&id=2125>.

10 Journalling

Adams, Kathleen. 'A brief history of journal writing'. *Center for Journal Therapy*, 1999. <http://journaltherapy.com/journaltherapy/journal-cafe/journal-writing-history>.

Baker, K.C. and Mazza, N. 'The healing power of writing: Applying the expressive/creative component of poetry therapy'. *Journal of Poetry Therapy*, 2004; 17(3): 141–54.

Capacchione, Lucia. 'Guidelines: Just a few tips before you begin creative journaling'.   <www.luciac.com/index.php/2012-10-21-20-32-30/the-art-of-finding-yourself/103-guidelines-just-a-few-tips-before-you-begin-creative-journaling>.

Center for Journal Therapy. 'Journal writing: A short course'. <http://journaltherapy.com/journaltherapy/journal-cafe/journal-course>.

Grason, S. *Journalution: Journaling to Awaken Your Inner Voice, Heal Your Life and Manifest Your Dreams*. New World Library, Novato, CA, 2005.

Pennebaker, James W. 'Disclosing and sharing emotion: Psychological, social and health consequences', in M. S. Stroebe, W. Stroebe, R. O. Hansson and H. Schut (Eds) *Handbook of Bereavement Research: Consequences, Coping and Care*. American Psychological Association, Washington, DC, 2001.

Pennebaker, James. 'Writing and health: Some practical advice'. <http://homepage.psy.utexas.edu/homepage/Faculty/Pennebaker/Home2000/WritingandHealth.html>.

Schlosberg, Paul. 'Personal growth journaling blog'. <www.createwritenow.com/personal-growth-journaling-blog/bid/51559/mindful-journaling>.

11 Mindful relationships

Cloud, H. and Townsend, J. *Boundaries*. Zondervan, Grand Rapids, MI, 1992.

Gillissen, Wendy. 'Dealing with hypersensitivity: The "secret" to not suffering from other people's feelings'. <http://ezinearticles.com/?Dealing-With-Hypersensitivity---The-Secret-to-Not-Suffering-From-Other-Peoples-Feelings&id=3114914>.

Grossman, D. 'Don't let fear destroy your relationship'. *PsychCentral*, November 2012. <http://psychcentral.com/lib/2011/dont-let-fear-destroy-your-relationship/>.

Hendrix, H. *Getting the Love You Want*. Harper & Row, New York, 1988.

Narcissism Support Resources. 'Narcissism symptoms'. <http://narcissism-support.blogspot.co.uk/2009/01/narcissism-symptoms.html>.

Orloff, J. *Emotional Freedom: Liberate Yourself from Negative Emotions and Transform Your Life*. Three Rivers Press, New York, 2011.

Rosetree, R. *Empowered by Empathy*. Women's Intuition Worldwide, Sterling, VA, 2001.

Young, J. *Cognitive Therapy for Personality Disorders: A Schema-Focused Approach*, 3rd ed. Professional Resources Press, Sarasota, FL, 1999.

12 Creativity, work and dreams

Anxiety Disorders Association of America. 'National stress out week highlights stress management in the workplace'. <www.adaa.org/about-adaa/press-room/press-releases/national-stress-%C3%B8ut-week-highlights-stress-management-in-the-workplace>.

Aron, Elaine, E. *The Undervalued Self*. Little, Brown, New York, 2010.

Boden, M. *The Creative Mind: Myths and Mechanisms*. Routledge, New York, 2003.

Dunning, D. *What's Your Type of Career? Find Your Perfect Career by Using Your Personality Type*. Nicholas Brealey Publishing, Boston, MA, 2010.

Talent Development Resources. 'Distracting ourselves from creative work'. <http://talentdevelop.com/5930/distracting-ourselves-from-creative-work/>.

Tieger, P. D. and Barron, B. *Do What You Are: Discover the Perfect Career for You Through the Secrets of Personality Type*. Little, Brown, New York, 2007.

Keirsey, D. *Please Understand Me II: Temperament, Character, Intelligence*. Prometheus Nemesis Book Co., Del Mar, CA, 1998.

Further reading

Aron, Elaine E. *The Highly Sensitive Person*. Birch Lane Press, New York, 1996.

Barlow, D. *Anxiety and its Disorders: The Nature and Treatment of Anxiety and Panic*. Guilford Press, New York, 2004.

Brantley, J. *Calming Your Anxious Mind: How Mindfulness and Compassion Can Free You from Anxiety, Fear, and Panic*. New Harbinger Publications, Oakland, CA, 2007.

Chozen Bays, J. *Mindful Eating: A Guide to Rediscovering a Healthy and Joyful Relationship with Food*. Shambhala Publications, Boston, MA, 2009.

Cloud, H. and Townsend, J. *Boundaries: When to Say Yes, when to Say No to Take Control of Your Life*. Zondervan, Grand Rapids, MI, 1992.

Dunning, D. *What's Your Type of Career? Find Your Perfect Career by Using Your Personality Type*. Nicholas Brealey Publishing, Boston, MA, 2010.

Ford, A. *The Art of Mindful Walking: Meditations on the Path*. Ivy Press, Lewes, UK, 2012.

Greenberger, D. and Padesky, C. *Mind Over Mood: Change How You Feel by Changing the Way You Think*. Guilford Press, New York, 1995.

Hendrix, H. *Getting the Love You Want*. Pocket Books, New York, 2005.

Jacobsen, M. E. *The Gifted Adult: A Revolutionary Guide for Liberating Everyday Genius*. Random House, New York, 2000.

Kabat-Zinn, J. *Full Catastrophe Living: How To Cope With Stress, Pain and Illness Using Mindfulness Meditation*. Piatkus, London, 2001.

Keirsey, D. *Please Understand Me II*. Prometheus Nemesis Book Co., Del Mar, CA, 1998.

Marks, I. *Fears, Phobias, and Rituals: Panic, Anxiety, and their Disorders*. Oxford University Press, New York, 1987.

Scott, T. *The Antianxiety Food Solution: How the Foods You Eat Can Help You Calm Your Anxious Mind, Improve Your Mood, and End Cravings*. New Harbinger Publications, Oakland, CA, 2011.

Wansink, B. *Mindless Eating: Why We Eat More Than We Think*. Bantam Books, New York, 2006.

Index